THE 30-MINUTE ANTI INFLAMMATORY DIET COOKBOOK FOR BEGINNERS

101 Easy-To-Cook Recipes to Reduce Inflammations | Stimulate Autophagy | Slow Down Skin Aging & More

Claire K. Mcloss, Dorothy Plumb

Table of Contents

Anti-Inflammatory Diet Cookbook

AUTOPHAGY: "SELF-MUTILATION" AS A SURVIVAL STRATEGY.................................... 15

CHAPTER 2: 5 Kitchen Staples That Everyone Should Have 25

CHAPTER 3: Mango Turmeric Lassi 31

CHAPTER 4: Snacks and sides recipes... 39

CHAPTER 2: 5 Kitchen Staples That Everyone Should Have 66

CHAPTER 3: Mango Turmeric Lassi 72

CHAPTER 4: Snacks and sides recipe 80

Anti-Inflammatory Diet for Beginners

Introduction 110

Chapter 1: What Is Inflammatory Disease 111

Inflammation and Overall Health: 113

Distinguishing Inflammatory Disease from Other Illnesses 116

Diagnoses of Inflammatory Disease and your Next Steps: 116

Chapter 2: Resolving Anti-Inflammatory Disease 121

Anti-Inflammatory Diet 121

Benefits of the Diet.. 124

Different types of food that are part of the Anti-Inflammatory Diet 125

Foods to avoid 128

Chapter 3: History of the Anti-Inflammatory Diet 131

Chapter 4: The Diet and You.. 134

Chapter 5: Tasty meals... 138

Chapter 6: Traveling with the Anti-Inflammatory Diet **145**

Mediterranean: 145

India: 148

Mexican/Hispanic Food/Latin: 150

Asian Food: 152

Italian: 153

Chapter 7: Setting Up A Schedule: Taking Action **157**

Sunday: 157

Monday: 158

Tuesday: 160

Wednesday: 161

Thursday: 163

Friday: 165

Saturday: 167

Chapter 8: The Popular Diet **169**

Mike Tyson: 170

Kevin Smith: 171

Penn Jillette: 171

Hannah Teter: 172

David Haye: 172

Barney Du Plessis: 172

Nate Diaz: 173

Meagan Duhamel 173

Gama Pehalvan: 173

Venus Williams: 173

Scott Jurek: 174

Jermain Defoe: 174

Ellen DeGeneres: 174

Usher: 174

Conclusion **176**

Description **177**

Anti-Inflammatory Diet Cookbook

An Easy Meal Plan for Beginners with Plant based, alkaline Diet and Autophagy to Heal The Immune System, Eliminate Inflammation, Lose Weight and Improve Your Health

DOROTHY PLUMB

DEACIDIFY, PURIFY - BE HEALTHY

Deacidification is one of the most critical steps on the way to health. How to properly deacidify the body, one believes long to know. And yet, after some acidification treatments, the results are not infrequent. The reason: Many deacidification treatments deacidify the gastrointestinal tract. But they do not deacidify the tissue, and they certainly do not deacidify the cell itself.

Deacidify and purify

Deacidification is a lifestyle today. Because deacidification is essential - at least when modern living and eating are modern. Ready meals, sausages, cheeses, snacks, sweets, soft drinks, caffeine, nicotine, and alcohol are now part of everyday life, but all of them acidify the organism. Similarly, environmental toxins, heavy metals, and poisons from textiles or building materials acidify. Stress, bullying, and strife eventually overflow the acid barrel called man. As a result, much and often, but not correctly, is deacidified.

Deacidification - an unfulfilled dream?

Usually, a healthy body can regularly deacidify and detoxify itself - without the human being having to intervene here. Today, however, the detoxification and purification capacities of the organism are often overburdened. And so the body can usually no longer neutralize on its own.

For autonomous deacidification, he lacks the basic requirements of a healthy lifestyle such as exercise, sunlight, micronutrients, relaxation, water, harmony, and - most importantly - an elemental diet. Deacidification, therefore, remains an unfulfilled dream for many people, and the acids and slags remain in the intercellular tissue. However, the intercellular fabric has the task of supplying and disposing of the cells.

One can imagine the intercellular tissue as a supermarket for the cells with the attached waste disposal plant. Cells receive everything they need from intercellular tissue: glucose, oxygen, vitamins, amino acids, fatty acids, minerals, etc.

At the same time, they permanently release their waste, including acids, to the intercellular tissue. The intercellular fabric is thus dependent on an agile transport mechanism. Nutrients and micronutrients must be produced, and waste must be transported away.

If not deacidified, the cell suffocates

If there is acidification, the intercellular tissue is used as a reservoir for acids and slags. This causes the river to falter. Waste can no longer be wholly removed and remains lying, which aggravates the acidification and slagging.

At some point there is hardly any room left for other waste, including acids. The cells do not know what to do with their garbage and have to store it in their interior. As a result, the cell itself now too acidifies.

In a sluggish intercellular tissue, of course, at the same time, the nutrient supply is at risk. For how should nutrients and micronutrients find their way to the cells when the intercellular tissue is full of slags and acids? Not only does the cell suffocate almost from its waste, but it also hardly receives the much-needed nutrients.

The cell lives like a slum. She is hungry and surrounded by garbage. Understandable, when she gets angry.

Acidification makes you sick and ugly

But slurred and over-acidified intercellular tissue, together with malnourished and acidic cells, is the prerequisite for everything we really do not want:

- overweight
- cellulite
- varicose veins
- Spider veins
- Impure or gray skin
- hair loss
- brittle fingernails
- joint pain
- Dental and gum problems
- bad eyes
- Lack of concentration and much more
- Deacidification makes you healthy and attractive

What we would like to have would be here:

- ideal weight
- Smooth and flawless skin
- Healthy blood vessels
- Full and healthy hair
- Strong fingernails
- Movable joints
- Healthy teeth until old age
- Sharp view
- Ability to concentrate and many more positive things
- Magic word deacidifying the body

Deacidification is the magic word. This is nothing new anymore. Therefore half of the world is currently deacidified - mostly in the following way:

A base powder is used to provide the organism with sufficient minerals that it needs to neutralize the acids that accumulate and to provide the resulting slags for disposal.

Base baths are used to excrete slag and acids through the skin. Also, brush massages are performed to stimulate deacidification via the lymph.

It turns the diet on a basic diet, avoid acidifying foods, and preferably alkaline foods. Here is a list of sour and alkaline foods.

It is dedicated to moderate exercise.

You try to avoid stress.

If deacidification fails

Of course, these measures are already outstanding. Nevertheless, success is too often limited or even completely absent. Why? At points 2 to 5, there is nothing to complain about. They not only support effective deacidification but are also a prerequisite for preventing further unwanted acids from entering the body. But there are two serious problems that prevent deacidification.

Deacidification requires basic nutrition

Problem 1: The diet is usually only slightly changed. On the one hand, because habits are difficult to change. On the other hand, because the right information and the right motivation are missing. Special detoxification treatment is ideal for getting into the right base excess diet. With such a detoxification cure over four weeks, you can easily learn to change your eating habits and receive a variety of suitable recipes.

You can feast basically

Find out more about the varied basic breakfast and get to know the healthy deacidified alkaline cakes. Experiment with basic spreads, basic potato dishes, and basic snacks. Immerse yourself in the basic world of crisp, healthy sprouts. And if you want to get to know the ultimate in basic lifestyles, then you should learn about green smoothies.

Deacidification requires high-quality base preparations

Problem 2: However, the measures mentioned above alone are often not enough to successfully deacidify. In many cases, they no longer manage to deacidify the organism and especially the cell interior. For this reason, a base preparation (point 1) is always prescribed for deacidification cures. And here - in the quality of the base preparation - is the reason for unsuccessful Entsäurerungskuren hidden.

Acidification of the cells

Many base preparations often deacidify only the gastrointestinal tract, but not the tissue and not the cell itself. And so the slag and many acids remain largely in the body. The hyperacidity does not only take place in the gastrointestinal tract, where it can be relatively easily neutralized with the mentioned minerals. Hyperacidity also takes place directly in the cell - with devastating effects.

You have to know:

A basic (= healthy) cell is negatively charged.

An acidified (= sick) cell is positively charged.

As with iron magnets with north and south poles, it behaves with electromagnetic charges: same poles/charges repel each other, different poles/charges attract.

The nutrition of the cell takes place by electromagnetic means.

Nutrients that the cell needs are positively charged.

If the cell is basic = healthy = negatively charged, it can attract nutrients and thus feed and produce energy.

If the cell is acid = sick = positively charged, it repels nutrients, so it can no longer feed, can not produce energy, the body decays.

An acidic cell can be given as much base powder or nutrients as you want - it simply can not absorb the minerals or nutrients. Deacidification does not take place; a therapeutic success remains.

Deacidify the cell

However, there is a way out. The cell can now be quickly and effectively freed from its acid reaction rigidity and converted into a basic living state - with the alkaline active water concentrate active bases.

In addition one must know again:

The positive charge of an acidified cell is due to a high concentration of H + ions.

Water (H2O) is a molecule and consists of 2 hydrogen atoms (2 times H) and 1 oxygen atom (1 time O), hence the name H2O.

Now you can also convert water into an ionic form. For this, one needs strong electric current, salt, and other special technological conditions. Then, you get positively charged H + ions (per molecule of water) and negatively charged OH - ions (also per molecule of water). This is still water, but it now has a lot of electrical potentials and ... it's very basic.

Deacidification with active bases

The name of this water is "active bases." If you drink this water, then these H + and OH - ions float around in the intercellular tissue, ie, in the fluid that surrounds the cells. The positively charged H + ions are repelled by the positively charged, but acidified cell, but the negatively charged OH ions are attracted and can enter the cell.

Deacidify every single cell

And now the fascinating thing happens:

Part of the penetrating negative OH ions combines with the positive H + ions (which are inside the cell) to form water. The other part brings the cell into a negatively charged, ie, basic state. The newly created water now flooded the accumulated garbage out of the cell, while the cell at the same time by the negative charge again nutrients attract and can also absorb, because only now - since the garbage was taken out - even more, space for nutrients.

The cell no longer has to live in filth and hunger. She is well looked after again and clean around her. The gloomy slum became a pretty residential area.

Deacidified with active bases

Active Basen is a concentrate with a pH between 10.5 and 11. Therefore it is taken in small amounts and diluted with water.

Directions for use: Twice a day, add 25 milliliters in about 150 milliliters of water (which is a small glass), and drink about 1 hour before a meal.

Deacidification with active bases should be carried out purely prophylactically twice a year. In case of complaints more often, in order to give the cells sufficient opportunity actually to leave the acidic state of the reaction rigidity.

Learn now how to properly and successfully deacidify. We will also introduce you to four acidification treatments - the right one for every person, every condition, and every everyday life. Two of them are based on active bases and are especially recommended for those people who have been acidified for a long time and finally want to find a way out:

The deacidification program

Carry out a 1 to 3-month deacidification program, e.g., B. with basic active water concentrate (active bases). These programs allow both extra- and intracellular deacidification. As part of a high-quality deacidification treatment - depending on the selected cure - you will be accompanied by other components that accelerate and intensify the deacidification. Basic baths, bitter substances, liquid bentonite, basic tea, etc.

If you find that the daily time spent on such a complete program seems too high, but you still want to deacidify, then you can opt for the simplest, yet successful method of deacidification with active bases. Active Basen is a basic active water concentrate that can deacidify the body down to the cell level. In the case of acid-base deacidification, you only have to think about taking active bases twice a day. That's all.

Eat base excess - even AFTER your 1 to 3-month detoxification treatment. The cure was only the entry! Those slags that have been in your body for many years can often only be eliminated after several months of basic life. In addition, you must also consistently withdraw the always new incoming acids or those that result from mental or physical stress.

If you still want to eat acidifying unhealthy food now and then, you must regularly provide your organism with high-quality alkaline minerals (e.g., a vegetable base powder, a citrate mix, or the Sango Marine Coral) to remove as many acids as possible can. Any change towards a healthy diet increases the chances of daily complete slag disposal.

Include the following points (or at least some of them) in your future daily routine:

Start the day with a basic morning tea.

Use basic body care products as basic as possible (see basic body care, e.g., a basic shower gel, a basic shampoo, etc.)

If you are in a hurry in the morning, have breakfast with a quick-prepared based cereal.

To supplement your diet with high-quality basic substances, you can sprinkle a vegetable base powder over each meal.

Organic basic minerals such. For example, the Sango Marine Coral is regularly ingested so that the body can finally return all the minerals it has borrowed from its mineral deposits during the depletion.

Relax at least two to three times a week in a base bath. If you do not have time for a full bath, you should treat yourself to basic foot baths.

Pay attention to deep, conscious breathing.

Plan moderate sports and sauna visits in your weekly routine.

In the evening you enjoy basic evening tea.

In natural medicine, it is also assumed that you can also deacidify well on the soles and therefore recommends base stockings that are worn at night and continue to deacidify in your sleep.

Check your deacidification success with the Sander acid-base test.

The acid-base test shows the degree of hyperacidity

Before a base therapy (deacidification), you can determine the degree of hyperacidity with the help of an acid-base test. In this way, it is much easier to assess whether and in what form deacidification is required.

WHAT IS AUTOPHAGY?
The body is not a rigid structure, but a highly complex and dynamic masterpiece. Construction and dismantling always take place in parallel, also parallel in the same line. The degradation can be done thoroughly; the utilization of carbohydrates and fats to CO_2, water, and energy in the form of ATP is known. The incomplete degradation of complex molecules into the individual components is often overlooked:
During autophagy, the cell degrades parts of the cell interior is tiny drops of fat (vesicles), and from them, extracts new building blocks (amino acids, sugars, nucleotides,).
These fat droplets are referred to herein as autophagosomes.
The term *autophagy* is composed of *auto* (Greek for self) and phagocytosis ("cell eating"). Colloquially, the cell partly eats/digests itself. However, this has little to do with suicide,

more with recycling: Autophagy contributes to the breakdown of old and damaged cell components and is essential for keeping the cell young and vital 1,9.

Autophagy is possible in every single cell in the body, but it also takes place outside the battery in the immune system : In fasted states in which autophagy is activated, macrophages circulate throughout the body, increasingly looking for infected cells, dead cells and pathogens, If you are sick in bed with flu, your body suppresses feelings of hunger to activate autophagy, which helps fight the infection.

A special form is a pinocytosis: This instrument, also known as "cell-drinking," is used by the cell to absorb, recycle, and self-use new cell material from lymph in large quantities.

Autophagy translates with self-digestion. It refers to a process in living cells in which cell components are broken down and utilized. At least 35 genes control the complex regulated process. For many decades, the autophagy has been explored by, among others, the Japanese molecular biologist Yoshinori Ohsumi. In October 2016, he received the Nobel Prize for Medicine for his work.

The autophagy proceeds as follows: First, the cell lays a unique sheath around the components that are to be broken down. The sheath closes to the autophagosome. This then fuses with lysosomes; these are small bubbles full of enzymes. The enzymes have the ability to break down and break down the components included in the shell. For example, it creates amino acids and lipids that can be newly installed or used for energy. The body identifies other degradation products as waste; they have transported away and excreted.

Autophagy is mainly triggered when the supply of nutrients stops. A situation that arises, for example, during fasting or intense sports. In this situation of deficiency, the cell relies on its resources. It breaks down what is not needed and thus gains new nutrients and energy. For self-digestion, the body dissects dead cell components, faulty proteins, and even whole-cell organelles, such as older mitochondria. Even pathological or potentially pathogenic structures, as well as invading bacteria and viruses, are disposed of. Therefore, autophagy is often described as a process of self-purification and self-preservation. It has evolved in the course of evolution to eliminate defective structures while conserving energy and nutrients.

In contrast to the natural renewal of body cells and organs, autophagy is much faster and more flexible. It can provide cell renewal virtually daily, while a real rejuvenation of cells can take days to years.

Autophagy also plays a role in the fight against infections and stress, as well as in embryonic development, to quickly have the required building blocks ready. Since a temporary energy deficit favors autophagy, it can be activated by fasting. This is another explanation for the positive health effects caused by regular fasting.

AUTOPHAGY: "SELF-MUTILATION" AS A SURVIVAL STRATEGY

In nature, nothing is lost: both for living things and for the entire biosphere, processes are characteristic in which a large part of the starting materials is recovered. One such regulation of the human cell is autophagy - a recycling program that allows it to break down damaged or misfolded proteins down to whole organelles and then reuse them. The phenomenon of autophagy was first described in the 1960s; For a long time, only a small group of researchers devoted themselves to this area. This has changed in recent years. Now the importance of this important cell process is reflected in the Nobel Prize Committee's recognition: The Japanese Yoshinori Ohsumi is honored for his discoveries of autophagy mechanisms. His work "has dramatically changed the understanding of this vital process," says the Nobel Prize committee's rationale.

With the crucial experiments, Ohsumi started in the early 1990s on yeast cells (Saccharomyces cerevisiae). At that time, it was already known that certain organelles, the lysosomes, degrade cellular components. The Belgian Christian de Duve had already received the Nobel Prize in 1974. It was he who coined the term autophagy.

But it was not until Ohsumi's work that it became clear which processes were going to be exactly the same and how important they are for human health. With a series of sophisticated experiments, he showed that 15 genes are involved in autophagy. Using his research, he described the network of signals and proteins that control the process in its various stages.

Cellular recycling: a highly complex process

Recycling is a matter of course for cells - the molecular waste is precisely packed by a membrane and sent to the lysosomes for recycling. In this highly complex process (graphic)Cell components that are no longer performing their task properly are channeled into the interior of autophagosomes. These are vesicles with a double membrane, which include proteins, lipids, membrane components, and whole organelles (mitochondria) from the cytoplasm into their interior. The autophagosomes then merge with lysosomes to autophagolysosomes, where the particles are degraded by acid hydrolases, and their basic building blocks are made available for recycling. Ultimately, this mechanism helps to keep the degradation of old and the production of new cell components in balance (cellular homeostasis).

Autophagy is continuously active at a basal level but is specifically activated in stressful situations. In extreme situations, such as severe cell damage, either apoptosis or so-called autophagosomal cell death - a non-apoptotic, programmed cell death - can be initiated. Autophagy is thus a mechanism for survival of the individual cell, but also a suicide program for damaged cells to ensure the survival of a multicellular organism. "It is therefore easy to understand that a dysregulated or diminished autophagic activity, as we presumably find it in old age, inevitably leads to a cellular disaster that manifests itself in a whole range of diseases.

These include:

- Cancer (lack of tumor suppression, dysregulated cell death, lack of elimination of damaged organelles),
- Accumulation of neurodegenerative plaques in dementia (impaired intracellular protein degradation),
- Muscular diseases (neuromuscular syndromes, myopathies),
- Infectious diseases (disturbed autophagosomal elimination of intracellular pathogens),
- functional hepatic insufficiency.

Autophagy: what do you have?

Autophagy plays a role, among other things, in the normal functioning of your immune system and in defence of (infectious) diseases. We will tell you more about the benefits of autophagy later in this post.

AUTOPHAGY: HOW DOES IT WORK?

As mentioned earlier, you can stimulate autophagy by doing a detox. More about that later. First autophagy. How does that work?

Your cells make membranes. These membranes look for dead or damaged cells in your body. Their goal is **to clean up** and reuse these **dead or damaged cells,** where possible. Membranes remove the good, yet to be used, parts from a cell and use these parts to make new cell parts.

That is how you clean up old cells in your body with autophagy. Autophagy makes our bodies better-oiled machines.

Autophagy is our body's way of **stopping dangerous cell division** and resolving issues such as obesity and problems with your metabolism.

ADVANTAGES OF AUTOPHAGY

There are many scientifically-proven benefits of autophagy.

1. CLEAN UP PROTEINS

Research shows that autophagy cleans up the proteins that may cause brain damage.

In certain brain disorders, proteins clump together in the body. Autophagy ensures that these clumps can no longer pose a threat.

The clumps are **surrounded by a kind of jacket** (autophagosome).

This jacket comes later with another jacket (lysosome) that is full of a digestive enzyme. The clumped proteins are thus rendered harmless.

2. LESS THICK AND BETTER BRAIN

There are indications that rats that are unable to autophagy are fatter and sleepier than their counterparts that are capable of autophagy. Also, they have higher cholesterol and a poorer brain.

- Supplying the cells with molecular building blocks and energy
- Recycling damaged proteins, organelles and aggregates
- Regulatory functions of the mitochondria of cells, which contribute to energy but can be damaged by oxidative stress
- Purification of damaged endoplasmic reticulum and peroxisomes
- Protecting the nervous system and promoting brain and nerve cell growth. Autophagy appears to improve cognitive function, brain structure and neuroplasticity.
- Support the growth of heart cells and protect against heart disease
- Strengthening the immune system by eliminating intracellular pathogens
- Protection against toxic proteins that contribute to a range of amyloid diseases
- Protecting the stability of the DNA
- Prevention of damage to healthy tissues and organs (so-called necrosis)
- Potential fight against cancer, neurodegenerative diseases and other diseases

THIS WILL GET MORE AUTOPHAGIA IN YOUR LIFE

It is good to know that autophagy is your body's response to stress. So to create some extra autophagy, you have to struggle through some stress.

1. SPORTS

Of course, you have known this for a long time; exercise causes stress. It is not for nothing that you puff and pant and moan and support during boat camps, weightlifting, running, Zumba and cycling.

Regular exercise is **the best way** that people unwittingly help renew their bodies.

A study among mice showed that the speed at which the creatures created autophagy increased after they had run on a treadmill for 30 minutes. The speed continued to increase until they were running for 80 minutes.

2. DETOXES

You are fasting with a detox; you do not eat periods. This can be stressful for your body. Your body may not like that at the time of the detox, but in the end, it benefits from this stress because you create autophagy.

Research shows that there are **many benefits of doing a detox,** also called periodic fasting. By regularly doing a detox, you help your body with autophagy.

Other research shows that fasting during a detox improves cognitive functions. Also, fasting would improve neuroplasticity (this helps your brain learn new things).

1. Fewer CARBON HYDRATES

By eating fewer carbohydrates, you relieve your body of its primary source of energy. Normally your body uses carbohydrates. By eating few carbohydrates (50 grams or less), you end up in ketose. Then your body uses fat as fuel instead of carbohydrates.

There are indications that ketosis can help people in **reducing the risk of diabetes.** Also, it is an ideal way to burn fat without losing muscle. For this reason, the ketosis diet is also very popular among bodybuilders.

What boosts autophagy in our cells?

1. Fasting (from about 14 to 17 hours, optimal are regular fasting treatment
2. Calorie restriction (chronic caloric deficit in a balanced diet)
3. Sport (both strength and endurance sports)
4. Some foods and substances: Grazer researchers have been able to identify foods and substances that turn on the cellular garbage disposal, even though the organism eats.

Coffee

Coffee, for example, is an autophagy trigger, the scientists confirm. The tasty pick-me-up is a very popular drink in Germany with a per capita consumption of around 5.5 kg a year. Studies show that coffee has extremely positive effects on various metabolic diseases, such as diabetes or lipid metabolism disorders.

Within one to four hours after the consumption of coffee, there is a strong stimulation of autophagy in all organs examined. This also applies to decaffeinated coffee, that is, it is not due to caffeine, but it is believed that phytochemicals, so-called polyphenols in coffee, have this effect. But beware: animal protein inhibits autophagy again, so do not put cow's milk in the coffee! Only black or with a herbal alternative such. B. Almond milk, coffee promotes self-cleaning of the cells.

WHAT CONTROLS AUTOPHAGY?

Cells do not just eat themselves. This process takes place only under very specific conditions and depends on complex molecular conditions. It involves enzymes such as mTOR and AMPK, which closely monitor how many nutrients and how much energy the cell has available. If there is not enough, they initiate the process of autophagy to break down old cell components that are not currently needed. The resulting components can then be used by the body to build up new and much-needed cell components.

By burning such contaminated sites into usable energy, the body can also guarantee the cell's survival in low-energy phases.

WHAT ARE THE TASKS OF AUTOPHAGY?

1. Autophagy as a survival mechanism

Digesting superfluous waste and using it as a building material or energy → Autophagy serves as a survival mechanism in barren times. Age researcher and Prof. Frank Madeo describes this process in a **lecture on youtube as** follows: "When cells are exposed to food shortages, they digest everything that is not needed, Cells are able to convert this "cell debris" into energy, which they then re-supply to the body. "

2. Autophagy as part of the immune system and defence mechanism

When foreign proteins or unwanted viruses and bacteria invade the cells, they are simply eaten up by autophagy and rendered harmless.

3. Autophagy as a cleaning-repair mechanism

In the many metabolic processes in our body, it always comes back to damage to cell components and the formation of defective proteins. To prevent them from causing any problems, autophagy simply breaks them down and eliminates them, which in the final stage can also lead to cell death, the so-called apoptosis.

When this purification process is disrupted, more and more substances are deposited in our cells, which is considered to be one of the main causes of cell ageing. One could also say that together with apoptosis, autophagy is the cellular quality control and therefore, essential for maintaining our functionality cells.

In animal experiments, it was shown that calorie reduction increases life expectancy. The reason could be the resulting increased autophagy, through which the cell components are broken down and rebuilt more often so that less "ballast" deposits.

When will autophagy be triggered?

Autophagy occurs to a lesser extent in all cells in the background but is exacerbated by food shortages (especially amino acid deficiency) and any other type of stress (metabolic, genotoxic, infectious and hypoxic).

So that means fasting and longer periods without food can start the process of autophagy. Researchers have found that we do not have to go hungry for days, but it's enough to fast for 14-18 hours a day, so-called **intermittent fasting.**

During this time, you should refrain from the intake of calories. Drinking water, tea or unsweetened coffee, however, is allowed. Coffee should even accelerate the onset of autophagy.

How to accelerate/amplify autophagy?

Autophagy can be accelerated by drinking coffee during the fasting phase. Apparently, it is not the caffeine that determines the supporting effect, but certain plant substances, so that caffeine-free coffee also works in this regard.

Also advancing autophagy is training during the fasting phase. There is no better way than fasting training to stimulate the purification process of the cells. The movement ultimately increases the energy requirement, and if this is not supplied from outside, cell waste can be particularly effectively recycled and burned to energy.

In addition, spermidine-containing foods such as wheat germ, fresh green pepper, mushrooms, soybean (especially fermented), citrus fruits (especially grapefruit) to promote autophagy.

On the other hand, overeating and high insulin levels inhibit the process of autophagy

- **supports autophagy:** long breaks between meals (keyword: intermittent fasting)
- calorie restriction
- Fast
- fasting training
- coffee
- spermidine-containing foods
- **inhibits autophagy too** frequent food
- high insulin levels (keyword: fast-digesting carbohydrates)
- animal protein
- Sugar, carbohydrates
- Too little movement

Is too much autophagy harmful?

After what has been said so far, it seems sensible to advance the process of autophagy. But autophagy can also be dangerous. In certain tumours, autophagy seems to accelerate the growth of cancer cells. Nevertheless, there is no reason for concern for the average consumer. Autophagy induced by fasting, calorie restriction, coffee, and other measures seems to have a positive effect on longevity and health.

THE PLACE OF AUTOPHAGY

The place of autophagy: this is how our cells are built

To understand the process of autophagy as far as possible, it is essential to get an overview of the structure of the cells.

Human cells are considered the smallest functional units of our organism. One can differentiate between cells with one cell nucleus (eucaryotes) and cells without a nucleus (prokaryotes). The typical human cell has a cell nucleus and consists of cytoplasm and the cell membrane as an outer shell. Among other things, the cell maintains its stability via this membrane. It also represents the gatekeeper for various substances. Some hold them back; others let them through into the cell interior. In this context, one speaks of the permeability of the cell.

The nucleus also contains the cell organelles. The nucleus, which is also called a nucleus, contains the genetic information in the form of DNA. A membrane, the nuclear membrane surrounds the cell nucleus itself. The cell organelle mitochondrion is of particular importance because it is considered the powerhouse of the cell. The cell membrane sets the starting point for autophagy, as it begins with certain signals through this recycling process. Another double membrane is created, which later starts with the inclusion of cell waste.

The autophagy in detail

It was the research of the Nobel laureate mentioned above that helped define the processes underlying autophagy. Among other things, the Japanese researcher was able to show that no fewer than 15 genes are involved in the process of autophagy. This also underscores the importance of self-cleaning of cells. The process control of these complex repair measures in the cell takes place, in turn, using specific proteins and signaling substances, which control every single step of the down-conversion process.

The cell begins to move no longer appropriately functioning cell components into the interior of the so-called autophagosomes. The latter is the dual-membrane vesicles already indicated above, which are capable of entrapping proteins, fats, other membrane constituents, or even mitochondria as a whole from within the cytoplasm in their interior.

Like waste in a garbage truck, faulty cell components are shunted into the autophagosome.

Autophagy is part of extensive cellular homeostasis because it helps balance essential cell components. In the process of fusion, autophagosomes, together with lysosomes, develop autophagolysosomes. In this process, the non-functional particles are broken down and converted into building blocks that can be recycled.

The possibilities of autophagy extend to cell death, which is referred to as autophagosomal cell death in comparison to apoptosis or programmed cell death. This cell death is caused by intense stress situations and intense cell damage.

That means autophagy for your health!

Many physicians believe that decreased activity in autophagy increases the risk of certain diseases. These include diabetes, cancer, neurodegenerative diseases, muscle diseases, infectious diseases, and hepatic insufficiency.

The decline in autophagic activity is increasingly associated with aging processes. You can imagine that the cells "waste." So if you want to avoid severe illnesses in old age, you must necessarily ensure that the "garbage collection" in the cells continues to work well and activate autophagy regularly.

This raises the question of how this can be done effectively.

With these tricks, the recycling program of the cells is stimulated!

Some scientists have long been concerned with the question of how to relieve flagellated autophagy. The current state of research highlights the following measures:

Interval fasting.

In particular, targeted periods of hunger, as can be achieved through fasting, are increasingly becoming the focus of interest.

Food with resveratrol.

Substances that mimic the biochemical processes of Lent will also help. The speech is, for example, of resveratrol. Studies have shown that this secondary plant substance from raspberries, grapes, plums, or red wine can also trigger autophagic processes in the cell. Another study even showed a connection between resveratrol and the prevention of Alzheimer's disease.

Food spermidine.

Another natural substance, spermidine, also acts on the activation of autophagy. The content is found, among other things, in various foods, such as in soy products, legumes, mushrooms, mature cheese, and wheat germ. Among other things, studies with fruit flies have shown that adding spermidine to food can counteract age-related dementia. It has also been demonstrated in an animal model with mice that the additional intake of spermidine protects heart health can. Background of the protective effects of spermidine is always that autophagic processes are intensified.

What does that mean for your body?

The cells stay healthier and, thus, the entire organism when the "garbage collection" in the cell is working correctly. It is still too early to make a final assessment of this, but there are many indications that most degenerative diseases are also the result of a tedious recycling function in human cells. As a result, both pathogens and degenerate cell components can accumulate, which over a long period causes loss of function and disorders at higher levels of the organism. Perhaps degenerative processes are, therefore, nothing other than the consequence of a disturbed renewal at the cellular level.

AUTOPHAGY ENDOGENOUS RECYCLING

Cellular building blocks for autophagy

The cells are fundamental building blocks of the organism. They are always busy developing, renewing, and multiplying. To understand how autophagy works in detail, it is essential first to understand the structure and operation of these small powerhouses.

Lysosomes - Decomposition of old and building new macromolecules

Not only in the household, but also on every level of the body must be regularly disposed of the garbage. Cells are confined to the outside by a plasma membrane. Inside is the so-called cytoplasm. This cytoplasm is watery in consistency and forms the carrier for the nucleus and various organelles such as lysosomes, mitochondria, and ribosomes. A membrane also encloses the lysosomes and contains different enzymes called acid hydrolases. These are responsible for the breakdown of fats, sugars, proteins, and nucleic acids within the cell. By dissecting and releasing these complex molecules, new macromolecules can be built up. Therefore, the lysosomes are often called the "recycling plant of the cell" designated.

Ribosomes take over the protein synthesis

The ribosome is composed of a complex combination of proteins and ribonucleic acid. In the ribosomes, protein synthesis takes place. In this case, individual amino acids are converted into long-chain polypeptides.

A ribosome represents a self-sufficient production facility for every protein to be synthesized in the body.

Mitochondria - power plants of the cells

The mitochondria are among the best known cellular building blocks. They are often referred to as "power plants of the cells" and responsible for the energy supply of the organism.

To maintain the body's substance, the cells must maintain an active metabolism. Metabolism means the construction, delivery, and degradation of proteins, carbohydrates, fats, and nucleic acids. The mitochondria supply the necessary energy for this. However, as these are not always available indefinitely, the cells must use this resource sparingly.

In the course of evolution, they have developed a technique to disassemble all available organelles or proteins into their parts completely.

It is a self-digestion process, which causes the decomposition of products to be re-metabolized. This process of recycling is the actual autophagy.

You can simplify the process by imagining a cleansing squad that swirls throughout the body, sweeping up any damaged or unneeded proteins, viruses, bacteria, cell organelles, plaques, and other microorganisms.

When this "heap" is complete, everything is burned and transformed into vital energy. Here, a healthy balance must be maintained in this perfectly coordinated mechanism.

In a figurative sense, exaggerated cleaning would cause cell death, while disruption or incomplete cleanup can trigger serious diseases such as cancer, Alzheimer's, or Parkinson's.

CHAPTER 2

5 Kitchen Staples That Everyone Should Have

Every healthy kitchen should always have these important things at hand.

1. nutritional yeast

It may seem intimidating at first, but it's nothing to be afraid of! This inactivated yeast is a powerhouse of nutrients that provides a great source of protein, B vitamins, folic acid, zinc, iron, magnesium, and the list goes on. It has a savory, nutty, cheesy taste and tastes great with salads, popcorn, vegetables, pasta, and soups.

2. Raw almond butter

Almond butter can help lower cholesterol, keep you full for longer, control blood sugar, and support weight loss (despite healthy fats!).

3. Chia seeds

These magical seeds work wonders in the body. Soaked in liquid, they take up nine times their weight, which means they form a jelly-like texture. These energizing seeds have twice as much protein as all other seeds, five times as much calcium as milk, twice as much potassium as bananas, three times as much iron as spinach, and a large amount of heart-healthy omega-3 and omega-6 fatty acids. Mix these seeds in your morning smoothie or make a delicious chia seed pudding!

4. Lenses

Lentils make a filling lunch or dinner and have an unlimited shelf life. Lentils are high in fiber, iron, B vitamins, and protein. The combinations are endless: lentil soup, lentil salad, lentil burger, lentil curry.

5. sea vegetables

This is the same kelp used for sushi. It has been found that Nori significantly reduces breast cancer risk and cholesterol levels. Not only is Nori used for sushi, but it is also great for making salad wraps, vegetable buns, or seaweed salad!

Hazelnut And Almond Macaroons

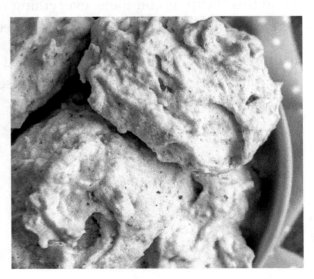

- 140 g protein (from about 4 eggs size M)
- 60 g of granulated sugar
- 130 g of powdered sugar
- 90 g of chopped hazelnuts
- 90 g of ground almonds
- 40 g almond flakes
- 1 pinch of cinnamon
- 1 pinch of salt
- Mark a vanilla pod

Roast the almond flakes lightly in a frying pan without fat and allow to cool. Put chopped hazelnuts, almonds, ground almonds, cinnamon and vanilla in a small bowl and sift the icing sugar. Preheat the oven to 145 ° C (top and bottom heat).

Beat the egg whites in a clean mixing bowl first on a medium, then on the fastest stage until frothy but not yet stiff. Add salt and granulated sugar, then beat until stiff. The egg whites should shine and stand on the turned whisk in firm tips upwards.

Carefully lift the powdered sugar and nut mixture in three portions with a spatula under the egg whites. Place the mass on a grid covered with baking paper with the help of two tablespoons and bake on the middle rack for 40-45 minutes. Allow the macaroons to cool, then carefully remove from the baking paper and store in a tight metal box.

Lemon dressing

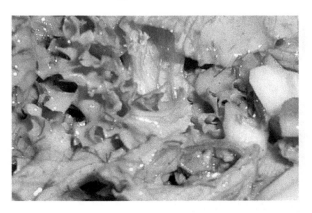

ingredients For

- 6 tbsp lemon juice
- 1 tbsp Lemon (s) - Peel, finely sieved
- 1 tbsp Mustard (Dijonsenf)
- 1 tbsp sugar
- 200 ml Olive oil, (not extra virgin)
- salt and pepper

preparation

Mix the lemon juice, peel, mustard, sugar, salt and pepper with the whisk, then slowly add the oil while stirring until the dressing has a creamy consistency. Goes well with crustaceans, fish, vegetables and fine lettuce.

Paleo Caesar Dressing

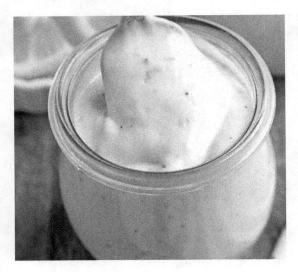

INGREDIENTS

- 2 eggs room temperature
- 1 ounce anchovies 1/2 can or about 5 filets
- 2 cloves garlic*
- 1/2 teaspoon salt
- 1/2 teaspoon pepper
- 1 tablespoon coconut vinegar or apple cider vinegar
- Juice of 1 lemon
- 2 - 2 1/2 cups light olive oil

INSTRUCTIONS

In a large mouth mason jar, combine eggs, anchovies, garlic, salt, pepper, vinegar, and lemon juice. Using an immersion blender, blend until completely smooth. About 30 seconds.

With the blender on, slowly pour in olive oil and move blender up and down in the jar until all oil is added and mixture is thick.

Aioli

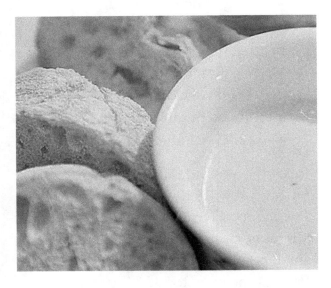

ingredients For

- 3 toe / n garlic
- egg yolk
- 250 ml Oil, neutral (eg sunflower oil)
- 1 teaspoon lemon juice
- salt and pepper

preparation

Place warm egg yolk in a bowl.

Peel garlic and process into a mortar in a mortar. Always add salt to make the paste bind. Then mix in a bowl with the egg yolk and a dash of lemon juice.

Add oil slowly, first drop by drop, later in a thin stream, whipping vigorously with the whisk all the while.

Be careful, add the oil too fast, the mass will clot, ie the process of splashing will take time!

Finally, season again and, if necessary, season with salt and pepper.

Juicy apricot and redcurrant slices with pistachio pesto

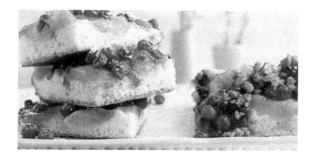

ingredients

- 1 kg of ripe apricots
- 500 g of redcurrants
- a little + 75 g soft butter
- 450 g + some flour
- 1 packet of baking soda
- 125 g + 1 tbsp sugar
- 1 packet of vanilla sugar
- salt
- 100 ml of milk
- 100 ml of oil
- egg (size M)
- 250 g of low-fat quark
- organic lime
- 100 g pistachios
- powdered sugar

preparation

Wash apricots, halve, stone and cut into wide slices. Carefully wash currants and brush with a fork from the panicles. A fat pan (deep baking sheet, about 32 x 39 cm) grease well.

Preheat oven (electric cooker: 200 ° C / circulating air: 175 ° C / gas: see manufacturer).

For the dough mix 450 g of flour, baking powder, 125 g of sugar, vanilla sugar and 1 pinch of salt. Add milk, oil, egg and quark and knead with the dough hooks of the mixer. Roll out the curd oil dough on the drip pan.

Press edges and corners with floured hands.

Spread 75 g butter in little flakes on the pastry. Give apricots and redcurrants. Bake cake in hot oven for 30-35 minutes. Remove and allow to cool on a wire rack.

For the pesto wash lime hot, pat dry and rub the skin. Squeeze out lime. Chop pistachios, lime zest and 1 tbsp sugar in a universal shredder or chop with a large kitchen knife.

Stir in the juice. Cut cake into pieces, dust with powdered sugar. To give the pistachio pesto.

Romesco sauce

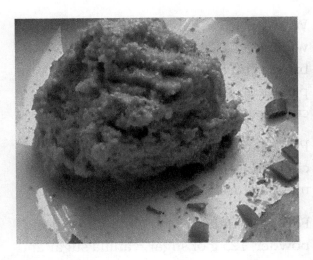

Put the tomatoes and peppers in the preheated oven and lightly toast for 1 hour at 150 ° C on baking paper, or better dry them so that the aroma and sweetness are better for the sauce. In the middle of the process, after half an hour, put the garlic cloves with the skin and roast.

Lightly toast the almonds and hazelnuts in a pan to enhance the aroma. Also goes in the oven but be careful not to burn them, go quickly.

Put the cooled paprika and tomatoes in a blender, remove the garlic from the skin and add to the tomato / pepper. Add the almonds and hazelnuts.

Then mix everything to a fine paste, mix the tomato juice, add the chilies cleaned and freed from the seeds.

The white bread with mix, the red wine vinegar and the olive oil, the red wine at the end of the sauce should be too thick with red wine or with oil to produce the desired consistency to taste.

ingredients

- 4 pcs of sun-ripened tomatoes
- 50 gr. Hazelnuts without skin
- 50 gr. Almonds without skin
- 4 garlic cloves
- 30 ml 30 ml olive oil cold pressed
- 3 tablespoons tomato juice
- 4 St. 4 chilis fresh & amp; quot; ancho & amp; amp; quot; and red
- 2 pieces of sliced toasted bread or breadcrumbs
- 1 tbsp red wine vinegar
- 1 tbsp red wine, dry and fruity
- 1 Msp. 1 Msp. Sea salt or to taste
- 1 Msp. Pimenton de la Vera or Paprika Rosenscharf
- 1 pc paprika red fresh

preparation

Remove the tomatoes from the stalk and slice.

Free the peppers from stalk and inner life and cut strips 2 cm.

Easy pasta pot with white beans

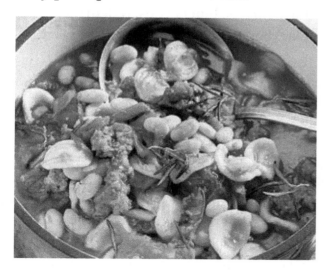

rosemary briefly. Add tomatoes, mince something. Pour 1 1/4 l of water, boil, stir in broth. Season with pepper and 1 tsp paprika. Add the pasta and simmer for about 18 minutes, stirring occasionally.

Rinse beans, drain. Heat in the last 2 minutes. Season with salt and pepper.

ingredients

- onion
- cloves of garlic
- branch rosemary
- 2 tbsp olive oil
- 300 g pig fat
- 1 tin (s) (à 850 ml) tomatoes
- 2 tablespoons vegetable broth (instant)
- pepper
- Sweet paprika
- salt
- 250 g small pasta (eg orecchiette)
- 1 tin (s) (à 425 ml) white bean seeds

preparation

Peel and dice the onion and garlic. Wash the rosemary, remove the needles.

Heat oil in a large saucepan. Roast Mett crumbly in it. Fry the onion, garlic and

Chapter 3:

mango turmeric lassi

ingredients

1 mango (about 350 g)

200 g skyr

2 Msp. Ground turmeric

2 tablespoons of agave syrup

1 tbsp lime juice

3 ice cubes (as you like)

preparation

Peel mango, cut into slices from the stone and roughly cut into pieces.

Together with skyr, 100 ml of water, turmeric, agave syrup, lime juice and if you want with ice cubes in a powerful blender to puree.

Would you like it more fluid? Mix another 1-2 tablespoons of water under the lassi.

Sweet fig smoothie

ingredients

2 cups of spinach fresh

5-10 raspberry leaves

1/2 avocado

1 cup of mixed fresh berries e.g. Raspberries, blueberries, redcurrants, blackberries

3 figs fresh

1 mango ripe

Juice of 2 oranges

instructions

Clean ingredients and cut to the size of the mix.

Halve the avocado, core it and remove the pulp!

Do everything in the blender and mix until smooth consistency!

Enjoy a fig smoothie from the heart!

Matcha berry smoothie

250 ml pear juice

125 g mixed berries

1 tsp honey

1 tbsp oatmeal

½ teaspoon matcha tea

That's how it's done:

Pear juice, mixed berries, honey, oatmeal and Matcha tea in the blender, mix well.

Ready is your smoothie!

Pumpkin Pie Smoothie

ingredients

135 g (½ cup) pumpkin from the tin

240 ml (1 cup) of milk

80 ml (⅓ cup) sweetened condensed milk

1 tablespoon of vanilla yogurt

1 teaspoon of pumpkin pie spice mixture

130 g (1 cup) ice cube

preparation

Put all ingredients into the Vitamix container in the order listed and seal with the lid.

Select setting 1.

Switch on the device, gradually increase the speed to level 10 and then up to "high".

Mix for 45 seconds or to the desired consistency.

Serve with whipped cream and a touch of cinnamon.

CARROTS PINEAPPLE GINGER SMOOTHIE

INGREDIENTS

3 carrots

15gr ginger

½ pineapple

1 banana

1 ½ limes

100ml of water

PREPARATION

So that the carrots can be mixed, you first peel the carrots. Then you throw them in a pot with a ground cover water, so they do not fry. Now they are cooked so that the carrots soften.

In the meantime you can halve the pineapple and cut out the pulp. Then you give the pineapple with the peeled banana and the juice of limes in the blender. You weigh the ginger and peel it. Give this with the now soft carrots together in the blender.

Now add some water and mix everything properly.

Apricot Cherry Tart with Frangipane:

For the dough:

60 g flour

60 g powdered sugar

2 tbsp powdered sugar

1/4 tsp salt

170 g cold butter, cut into small cubes

For the Frangipane:

65 g sugar

65 g soft butter

1 egg (size M)

100 g finely ground almonds

Scattered peel of 1 organic lemon

3 tablespoons milk or whipped cream

2 teaspoons flour

10-12 apricots, each cut in 6 columns

25-30 cherries, gutted and halved

Knead all ingredients together well for the dough and refrigerate for 1 hour in the fridge.

Preheat the oven to 190 ° C top and bottom heat.

For the Frangipane filling, stir the soft butter and the sugar until creamy. Then stir in the egg. Stir in the ground almonds, then the citrus peel and finally the milk or cream. Then stir in the flour briefly and quickly.

Press the dough into a greased Tart mold. Then fill in the Frangipane. Cover with apricot slices and cherry halves.

Bake the tart for about 35 minutes until the dough is golden brown. Remove and allow to cool.

apple spritzer

ingredients For

300 ml apple juice

1 splash Lemon juice, freshly squeezed

1 Cinnamon sticks)

Possibly. Sugar, brown, optional

preparation

Fill the apple spritzer with the lemon juice in a large glass. Put the cinnamon stick in the liquid, put the glass in the microwave. Heat at 800 watts for 2 minutes and 20 seconds.

Migas with Black Beans

INGREDIENTS

Crispy tortilla strips

4 small corn tortillas

1 ½ teaspoons olive oil

Salt

Spicy black beans (half of these peppers go into the eggs)

1 small red onion, chopped

1 red bell pepper, seeded and chopped

1 poblano pepper or 1 additional bell pepper, seeded and chopped

1 jalapeño pepper, seeded and chopped

4 garlic cloves, pressed or minced

2 teaspoons olive oil

1 teaspoon ground cumin

1 (15 ounce) can of black beans, drained

3 tablespoons water

Squeeze of lime juice or splash of sherry vinegar

Scrambled eggs

8 eggs

3 tablespoons cream or milk of choice

¼ teaspoon salt

Freshly ground black pepper

2 teaspoons olive oil

½ to ¾ cup grated Monterey Jack cheese or cheddar cheese

Garnishes

Chopped cilantro

Salsa and/or hot sauce of choice

More tortillas, warmed (optional)

Diced avocado (optional)

INSTRUCTIONS

Preheat oven to 425 degrees Fahrenheit and line a baking sheet with parchment paper while you're at it. Scramble 8 eggs with 3 tablespoons cream/milk, ¼ teaspoon salt and a few twists of freshly ground black pepper. Set the eggs aside for later.

Slice 4 tortillas into short, thin strips (see photos). Transfer the strips to your prepared baking sheet, then toss with 1 ½ teaspoons olive oil until lightly and evenly coated. Arrange them in a single layer and sprinkle with salt. Bake until crispy, flipping halfway, about 8 to 10 minutes.

Meanwhile, cook the pepper-and-onion mixture. In a medium saucepan over medium heat, warm 2 teaspoons olive oil. Add the chopped onion, bell pepper, jalapeño, garlic and a dash of salt. Cook, stirring often, until the onions are turning translucent and the peppers are tender, about 5 minutes. Transfer half of the mixture to a bowl for later and return the pot to heat.

To the pot, add 1 teaspoon ground cumin and sauté until fragrant, stirring constantly, about 30 seconds. Add the drained black beans and 3 tablespoons water. Stir to combine. Reduce heat to low, cover and simmer until you're ready to serve.

Once you have your crispy tortilla strips and reserved pepper mixture ready, you can scramble the eggs. In a 10-inch non-stick or well-seasoned cast iron skillet, warm 2 teaspoons olive oil over medium heat. Swirl the pan so it's evenly coated with oil. Add the peppers from your bowl to the skillet, then whisk your egg mixture one last time and pour it into the skillet.

Scramble the eggs by pushing the mixture around and 'round and 'round until they're about three-fourths set. Fold in the crispy tortilla strips and cheese and continue cooking until the eggs are scrambled to your liking. Remove from heat.

Remove the beans from heat. Use a fork to mash up about half the beans, then stir in a squeeze of lime or splash of vinegar. Season to taste with salt and pepper.

Divide migas and black beans into individual serving bowls/plates. Top with a sprinkle of chopped cilantro. Serve with salsa, warmed tortillas (optional) and diced avocado (optional) on the side.

Spinach and leek frittata

ingredients

spinach

250 g , spinach leaves (fresh or frozen)

Leek

1 pole (s), large , in thin strips

Chicken egg /

6 pieces

food starch

2 tsp

Milk, low fat, 1.5% fat

100 ml

Parmesan / Montello Parmesan

1 tbsp., Grated

sea-salt 1 pinch

pepper 1 pinch

manual

Preheat oven to 180 ° C. Place a baking tin, approx. Ø 20 cm, with parchment paper.

Blanch spinach in boiling water for about 2 minutes; drain and express lightly. Prepare TK spinach according to the package instructions. Chop cooled in rough strips.

Blanch the leek separately in 3 minutes; let drain, also express easily. Distribute both vegetables on the bottom of the baking pan.

Stir eggs, starch, milk and spices together; pour over the vegetables. Press the mass with a fork in the mold.

Spread the cheese over it, bake for about 18-20 minutes until the frittata has risen and is golden-brown.

10 min. allow to cool, remove the mold and serve cut into small pieces of cake.

Fried rice with egg

ingredients

600 g Rice, cooked

3 Egg (s)

½ Lemon (s), juice of it

thyme

Salt or soy sauce

pepper

oil

preparation

Heat pan or wok and let oil in it get hot. Add the cooked rice and stir-fry for a while, keeping it at the highest level. Season with pepper and salt or soy sauce, lemon juice and thyme. Whisk the eggs over and give, stir again really well, so that there are beautiful "Eierfetzchen". Season with pepper and salt or soy sauce.

Stir well after each ingredient, before adding the next one.

The length of the roasting time depends on the desired tan and consistency of the rice and the eggs. I always roast the rice for about 10 minutes, then come first the spices and the egg and then I let it fry as a whole again about 10 minutes.

Of course you can also vegetables (eg peppers or peas) or meat (but that should then make the roast) to give it, but it tastes best, even for breakfast or as a warm addition to the brunch.

Salmon trout on wild garlic puree with fried garlic

INGREDIENTS

Salmon trout fillet

Butter liquid for the wild garlic puree

6 big ones potatoes

Almond milk

salt and pepper

2 tablespoons Wild garlic chopped

plentiful butter

PREPARATION

first boil the potatoes soft - then peel and finely crush together with the almond milk, a little salt and pepper and wild garlic - ALTERNATIVE: my wild garlic comes at this time of year of course from the freezer, who has no wild garlic available, who could also use finely chopped rocket and some finely chopped garlic

Wash the fish, dab dry and remove all bones with tweezers - marinate with a little lemon juice - then brush with a brush lukewarm, liquid butter - brush a heat-resistant mold with the butter, put the fish on it, season with some sea salt and freshly ground pepper - Cook in the preheated oven at 120 degrees for approx. 14 minutes

bisect the garlic bulb in the middle - cut in a dry pan over medium heat while gently toasting the garlic cloves out of the shell ... the garlic gets very mild in the taste and almost a little sweet !!! tastes very fine !!!

Baked apple-Chia Pudding

ingredients

250 ml Soy milk (soy drink), (vanilla), alternatively another vegetable milk

4 tbsp Chia seeds

2 big ones apples

4 tbsp cane sugar

½ TL cinnamon

4 tsp raspberry jam

4 tbsp Walnuts, crushed

preparation

Let the chia seeds swell in the soymilk for at least 4 hours, preferably overnight.

Then make the baked apples. Peel the apples, core them and cut into small pieces. Add cane sugar, ground cinnamon, raspberry jam and crushed walnuts.

Put in the oven for 20 minutes at 200 ° C. Then let the baked apple pieces cool down a bit.

Now the whole thing is done. First, give the chia pudding in Gals. Then arrange the baked apple pieces on it - done.

Breakfast yoghurt with spelled sprouts

ingredients

70 g Sprouts (spelled sprouts, from approx. 40 g spelled grains)

150 g Natural yoghurt (3.8% fat) or natural soy yoghurt

1 tbsp Raisins, soaked

something Water for soaking

1 Msp. vanilla powder

1 m. -Large Apple

preparation

Drain the soaked raisins. Grate the apple with the shell and mix with the other ingredients.

Spelled sprouts are easy to grow from organic spelled grains. Soak the spelled for 12 hours and then germinate for 3 - 4 days. Rinse the germs twice daily. I prefer to use germination glasses for germination.

Spelled sprouts taste slightly sweetish (but not as sweet as wheat sprouts) and have a bit of a bite. In addition, spelled is rich in vitamin B3 (niacin), potassium and magnesium.

Healthy Banana Oatmeal Pancakes

ingredients For

1 cup Oatmeal, tender

1 Banana (s), ripe

1 Egg (s)

60 ml milk

1 teaspoon, heaped ground cinnamon

Something Butter for the pan

preparation

Crush the banana to a pulp with a fork or blender. Grind the oatmeal into flour, preferably with a flour mill, if necessary also with a blender.

Put all ingredients in a container. Purée until a smooth dough is formed. Put some butter in a small pan for frying and fry the pancakes in portions golden brown. For each serving, the recipe gives about 2-3 cakes.

As a side dish it tastes wonderful a bit of natural yoghurt with fresh fruit from the season. Optionally, but also with red groats, quark and banana pieces a treat.

CHAPTER FOUR

Snacks and sides recipes

Chinese eggplants

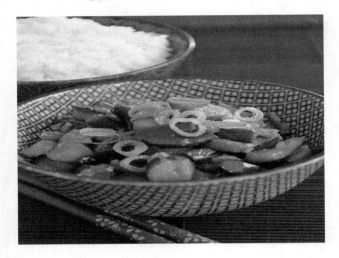

Ingredients *for 2 servings*

- 2 eggplants
- peanut oil or a neutral for frying
- 1-2 cloves of garlic
- 1 piece of thick piece of ginger
- 2 scallions
- 1 tablespoon sambal oelek
- 1 teaspoon sugar
- 2 tablespoons soy sauce
- 1-2 tablespoons rice vinegar
- Sesame oil for seasoning

Preparation

1. Peel the garlic and ginger and chop very finely.

2. Clean the spring onions, cut away the root and the dark, dry green and chop finely.
3. For the sauce, mix soy sauce, sugar, rice vinegar and Sambal Oelek with some sesame oil (for taste).
4. Wash, dry and dice the aubergines and sauté in very hot oil until they have a nice brown color on all sides.
5. Remove from the wok and mix with the sauce.
6. Add the garlic, ginger and spring onions to the remaining oil and fry gently. When a delicious scent develops, add the aubergines and sauce to the wok, mix well and fry for a few minutes.
7. A nice side dish to rice. Or just like that.

Simplest guacamole

Guacamole

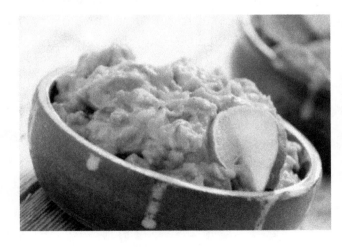

Ingredients *for 16 servings*

- 2 stk mild, red peppers
- 1 stk lime
- 2 stk ripe avocados
- spr Tabasco
- prize salt
- stk tomatoes
- prize Pepper (mill)
- stk small onion
- stk clove of garlic

Preparation

1 For this Mexican guacamole, first cut the peppers in half lengthwise, corer them and finely dice them. Peel the onion and cut into small pieces. Juice lime. Finely chop the tomatoes (it is best to add them to the boiling water, blanch , skin and core).
2 Then halve the avocados, remove the kernel and remove the pulp from the peel with a spoon - cut and slice avocados properly
3 Then puree the avocado meat and the lime juice (or lemon juice) in a blender.
4 Season the avocado puree with salt, pepper and Tabasco. Add the peppercorn cubes, onion pieces and diced tomatoes to the puree and let it steep for 15 minutes.

Spicy two-bean dip recipes

BEAN DIP

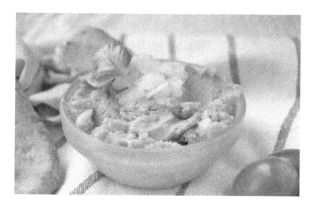

Ingredients *for 2 servings*

- 250G Beans (white)
- stk onion
- stk garlic
- EL butter
- TL tomato paste
- TL paprika
- prize Salt pepper
- shot olive oil

Preparation

1 Put white beans in water overnight or take them out of the can and wash thoroughly. Boil the beans in salted water until they are cooked. The beans are now mashed with a little boiled water.
2 Finely chop the onion and sauté in a pan with a little butter, add the pressed garlic clove, the beans and add the tomato puree. Pour some water if necessary. Turn down the heat.
3 Now season with the finely chopped parsley, salt, pepper, paprika and a dash of olive oil.

Simmer until it thickened nicely. Serve the dip with bread or something else for dipping.

Cashew hummus dip recipes

Cashew Hummus

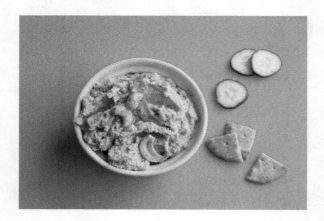

Ingredients

- 1 540-mL can chickpeas , drained and rinsed well
- 1/2 cup roasted, unsalted cashews
- 1/4 cup olive oil
- 1 tbsp fresh lemon juice
- 1/2 tsp finely chopped garlic
- 1/4 tsp ground cumin
- 1/4 tsp salt
- 3-4 tsp water

Preparation

1 Combine chickpeas with cashews, olive oil, lemon juice, garlic, cumin and salt in the bowl of a food processor. Purée until well combined.
2 Scrape down the sides of the bowl and continue blending, adding

water gradually until hummus is the texture you like.

Avocado-Apple-prosciutto wrap recipes

Avocado Ham Wraps

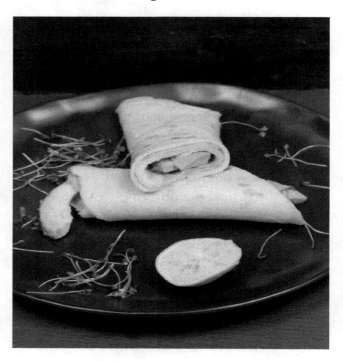

Ingredients

- 11/2 avocado
- slices of cooked ham
- 75 grams of wheat flour
- 25 grams of spelled wholemeal flour
- 1 pinch of salt
- 250 milliliters of milk
- 1 egg
- 1 teaspoon rapeseed oil
- 1 splash of lemon
- Freshly ground pepper

Preparation

1. Peel avocado and cut into slices. Drizzle with lemon juice.
2. Mix a pancake with flour, salt, milk and egg. Heat the oil in a non-stick pan and bake out 3 pancakes.
3. Cover each pancake with 2 slices of cooked ham and half an avocado. Peppers and then roll into a wrap. Cut to serve in the middle.

Roasted chickpeas Recipes

Roasted chickpeas

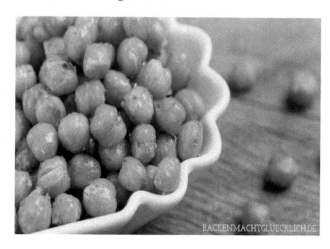

Ingredients

- cans of pre-cooked chickpeas per 250g drained weight; alternatively approx. 200g raw
- tablespoons of olive oil
- 1.5 tablespoons of sea salt
- 2 teaspoons paprika powder
- 1 pinch of chilli powder
- 1 pinch of garlic powder

Preparation

1. Drain the chickpeas from the tin, rinse and then dry or dab well. (Raw chickpeas must first be soaked overnight and then cooked for about 1.5 hours.) Preheat the oven to 190 degrees top and bottom heat. Cover a tin with baking paper.
2. Mix the dry chickpeas in a bowl with the olive oil. Spread on the plate and bake for about 25 minutes (depending on how crispy you want it or how your stove heats).
3. Twist or shake twice during the baking time to make the chickpeas brown evenly. Watch at the end of the baking time so they do not get too dark.
4. Remove from the oven, still hot with salt and spices and warm.

Salt & Vinegar Chips

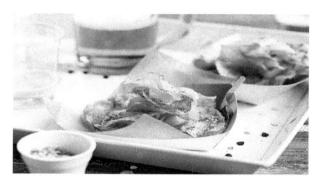

Ingredients for *2 servings*

- gold potatoes
- cups vinegar (480 mL)
- 1 tablespoon salt
- 1 tablespoon pepper

Preparation

1. Carefully slice 3 gold potatoes into ⅛ inch (3 mm) slices using a knife or mandoline.
2. In a large bowl, coat chips with vinegar so all are submerged, allow to sit for 30 minutes (the longer they sit the more vinegary they will taste).
3. Preheat the oven to 350°F (175°C).
4. Drain the chips and then mix in salt and pepper.
5. Arrange chips on greased baking sheet.
6. Bake for 30-35 minutes.
7. Enjoy!

Blueberry frozen yogurt recipes

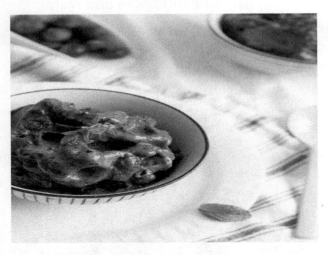

Ingredients

- 300 g blueberries frozen
- 150 g of yogurt at least 3.5% fat
- Sweetener and meringue to taste

Preparation

1. Puree frozen blueberries and yoghurt in a blender or with some stamina and a hand blender.
2. Fill in two bowls, lean back and enjoy.

Spicy avocado deviled eggs

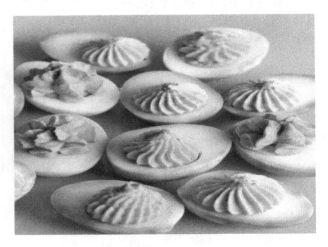

Ingredients *for about 8-10 egg halves*

Filling:

- 60 g organic salmon
- 60 g cream cheese
- 1 dash of lemon juice
- 60 g avocado
- 60 g cream cheese
- drops of lemon juice
- 100 g cream cheese
- 20 g pureed beetroot

- Salt / pepper
- Piment d'Espelette

For the colored eggs

- The broth from a
- large red cabbage, grated, boiled with a little water for 45 minutes.
- Juice of beetroot in the glass colored much stronger than my homemade puree
- 2 pieces of fresh turmeric, grated and boiled in 500 ml of water, the water is nice
- orange, remove the turmeric.

Preparation

1. Beat the hard-boiled eggs so that the shell is
2. cracked as evenly as possible. Place the eggs in each brew
3. and bathe in them for about 15-30 minutes.
4. No soda is first added to the red cabbage, some eggs are
5. dyed in it, and little bit of soda is gradually added until it reaches the
6. desired purple, blue and green shades.
7. Each salmon and avocado separately with the cream cheese with the
8. lightning hacker or blender puree and season with salt and pepper.
9. For the beetroot filling, add only so much puree that the
10. filling with the piping bag can be sprayed well, also season.
11. Fill all the fillings in the piping bag provided with the desired spouts
12. and either keep them cold or, when the eggs are completely
13. dyed, sprinkle them on.
14. Sprinkle all eggs with a pinch of Piment d'Espelette.
15. The eggs are still very handsome the next day, then discolored the avocado cream.

Sweet potato oat muffins

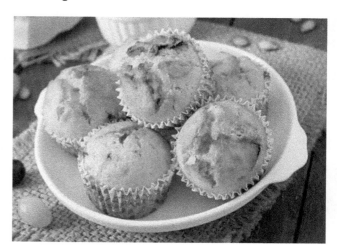

Ingredients

Dry ingredients:

- 150 g of ground oatmeal
- 75 g sugar of your choice
- 56 g of ground almonds
- 1/4 teaspoon soda
- pinch of salt

- 60 g milk-free chocolate chips and more for the top

Moist ingredients:

- 235 g of crushed sweet potato
- 160 ml of vegetable milk
- 1 tsp vanilla extract
- teaspoons vinegar

Preparation

1 Peel a medium sized sweet potato, cut into pieces / cubes and cook in water for about 10 minutes or until the pieces are soft (but not mushy). Drain the water and mash the sweet potato with a potato masher.
2 Preheat oven to 180 degrees C and lay a muffin dish with muffin paper or brush the inside of the molds with coconut oil. I used a silicone muffin mold.
3 Put all dry ingredients (except the chocolate chips) in a bowl and mix with a whisk. You can also process the dry ingredients in a sorler (I did that).
4 Add all wet ingredients and mix or mix in the Hexler until everything is mixed.
5 Finally, add the chocolate chips and stir with a spoon.
6 Spoon the dough into the muffin cups and spread more chocolate chips on top.

7 Bake in the oven for about 25 minutes or until a toothpick comes out clean. It's fine if the toothpick still comes out slightly sticky / crumbly, but it should not be wet.
8 Let the sweet potato muffins cool and enjoy!

Berry gummies Recipes

Currant butter cake from sheet metal

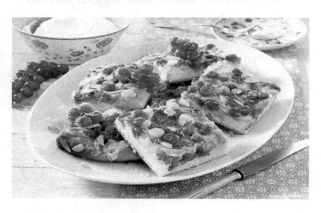

Ingredients *for 24 pieces*

- Fat and flour
- 200 ml of milk
- 1 cube (42 g) of fresh yeast
- 400 g of flour
- 75 g + 25 g + 2 tbsp sugar
- salt
- eggs (size M)

46

- 75 g + 225 g soft butter
- 500 g redcurrants
- 200 g of cold marzipan paste
- Flour
- 75 g almond flakes
- disposable syringe bag or small freezer bag

Preparation

1 Grease fat pan (about 32 x 39 cm, about 3.5 cm deep) and dust with flour. Warm the milk lukewarm. Break in the yeast and dissolve it. Mix flour, 75 g sugar, 1 pinch of salt, eggs and 75 g butter in little flakes in a bowl.

2 Add yeast milk and knead with the dough hook of the mixer. Cover in a warm place for about 45 minutes.

3 Read the berries, wash them and brush off the stems with a fork. Grate the marzipan roughly. Stir 225 g butter, marzipan and 25 g sugar creamy. Put in a disposable syringe bag.

4 Knead dough again. Dust with flour and roll out on the drip pan, pressing on the edge into the corners. Cover and let rise for about 20 minutes.

5 Press depressions into the dough with your thumbs or a thick wooden spoon. Cut off the tip of the piping bag. Spray marzipan paste into the wells. Distribute berries on the cake.

6 Sprinkle with almonds and 2 tablespoons of sugar. Bake in the preheated oven (electric cooker: 200 ° C / circulating air: 175 ° C / gas: see manufacturer) for 20-25 minutes. Allow to cool slightly.

Root mash recipes

Celery Root Mash

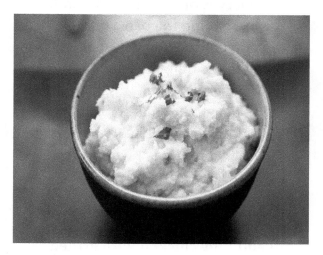

Ingredients

- pounds celery root
- 1/2 cup milk or cream
- tablespoons unsalted butter
- Salt to taste

- Chopped celery root leaves, for garnish (optional)

Preparation

1. Bring a large pot of salted water to a simmer (1 Tbsp of salt for every 2 quarts of water).
2. Peel and cube the celery root, boil until soft: While the water is coming to a boil, peel the celery roots with a knife. Cut the celery roots into 1-inch pieces.
3. Boil for 25-30 minutes, until soft.
4. Drain the pot, steam the celery root: Drain the pot, return the celery roots to the pot to the stovetop on low. Cover and let the celery roots steam for a minute or to, shaking the pan a bit to prevent sticking.
5. Add the milk or cream, butter and a generous pinch of salt and mash with a potato masher until it is as smooth as you like it. Add salt to taste and garnish with the celery root leaves, if using.

Lime-chili roasted cauliflower recipes

Chili and lime chicken with grilled sweet potato and cauliflower salad

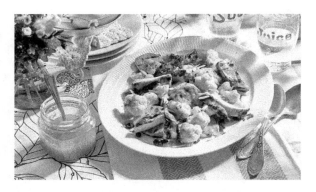

Ingredients *for 4 people*

- stalks / ciliary
- jalapenos
- cloves of garlic
- organic lime
- 1 tbsp and1 tsp liquid honey
- teaspoons and 1 pinch of salt
- 1 teaspoon chilli powder
- pieces (à 250 g) chicken fillet (with skin)
- 2 sweet potatoes
- small cauliflower
- 50 g almond sticks
- tbsp oil
- stalks / parsley
- 50 grams of almond paste
- 1 tablespoon of apple cider vinegar
- 1 teaspoon curry powder
- teaspoons of chilli sauce (eg Sriracha)
- pepper
- 50 g raisins

Preparation

1. Wash cilantro, shake dry. Peel leaves and chop finely. Wash, clean and finely chop jalapenos. Peel garlic and chop finely. Wash lime hot and rub dry. Rub the lime peel finely. Halve lime and squeeze juice. Juice, peel, coriander, jalapenos, garlic, 1 tablespoon honey, 2 teaspoons salt and 1 teaspoon chilli powder. Wash the meat, pat dry and mix with the marinade. Meat for about 2 hours.

2. Peel sweet potatoes, wash and cut into thin slices. Clean cauliflower, cut into small florets. Wash florets and drain well. Roast almonds in a frying pan without fat for about 3 minutes until golden brown and remove.

3. Heat 1 tbsp of oil in the pan. Cover with cauliflower and cook for 5-10 minutes. Then cook without lid for another 5-10 minutes until the cauliflower is golden brown.

4. Brush the grill with 1 tablespoon of oil, place the meat on the hot grill and cook until golden brown. Mix sweet potato slices and 2 tablespoons of oil. Place on the grill and grill on each side for 2-4 minutes until soft.

5. Wash parsley and shake dry. Peel leaves and chop finely. Almond flour, apple cider vinegar, 1 teaspoon honey, curry powder and chili sauce mix. Emplace 4 tbsp of oil. Season with salt and pepper. Remove meat and vegetables from the pan. Cut meat into strips. Serve meat, vegetables, almonds and raisins on plates. Sprinkle with parsley.

Cider-baked recipes

Frankfurt cider wreath

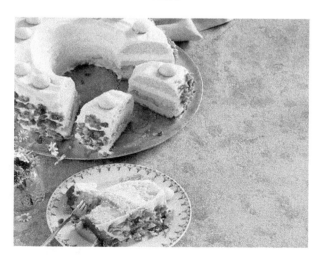

Ingredients *For 20 pieces*

- 200 g soft butter
- 1 tsp soft butter
- 1 pinch of salt
- 300 g of sugar
- tbsp sugar
- sachets of vanillin sugar
- eggs (size M)
- 225 g of flour
- 95 g cornstarch
- 1 packet of baking soda
- tablespoons milk
- sheets of gelatine
- apples
- Juice of 1 lemon
- 300 ml of cider
- 250 g of whipped cream
- 600 g double cream cream cheese
- 100 g dried soft apple rings
- Fat and breadcrumbs
- baking paper

Preparation

1 Mix 200 g of butter, salt, 200 g of sugar and 1 packet of vanillin sugar with the whisk of the hand mixer until creamy. Stir in eggs one after the other. Mix flour, 75 g of starch and baking powder and mix alternately with the milk under the fat-egg cream. Grease a ring mold (24 cm Ø, 2 liter content) well and sprinkle with breadcrumbs. Fill in the dough and smooth it out. Bake in preheated oven (electric cooker: 175 ° C / circulating air: 150 ° C / gas: see manufacturer) 35-40 minutes. Leave to cool on a wire rack for about 20 minutes. Drop out of the mold and allow to cool completely.

2 Soak the gelatine in cold water. Peel apples. Quarter 3 apples, cut out the core. Cut quarters into small pieces. In a pot with lemon juice and 150 ml of cider mix. Cover and simmer for about 5 minutes. Stir 50 ml of cider, 20 g of starch and 1 tbsp of sugar until smooth and stir in the compote, bring to a boil and allow to cool slightly.

3 Cut the cooled wreath 2x horizontally. Enclose lower bottom with a cake ring. Distribute the compote on top, place the middle of the tray and leave to cool for approx. 15 minutes. Whip the cream. Cream cheese, 100 ml of cider, 100 g of sugar and 1 packet of vanilla sugar mix. Express gelatin, melt. Stir in 1-2 tablespoons cream cheese cream, then stir in the remaining cream. Fold in the cream. Leave the cream for about 15 minutes until it gets a little firmer.

4 Stir again with cream and coat about 1/3 of the cream on the middle ground. Put on the upper

floor. Let it cool again for about 20 minutes. Remove the cake ring from the garland. Coat the wreath with the remaining cream all around. Cook the cake for about 2 hours. Dried apples cut into small cubes. Caramelise 4 tbsp sugar with 1 tbsp water in a small pan. Turn the apple cube into it and allow to caramelise for about 1 minute. Caramelised apples on a piece of baking paper, spread with the help of 2 forks and let cool.

5   Cut out balls from the rest of the apple using a ball cutter. Heat 1 tsp butter in a small pan, add apple balls, sprinkle with 1 tbsp sugar and deglaze with 1 tbsp water. Steam apple balls for about 2 minutes. Chop apple crisp small. Decorate cake with apple crisp and apple balls.

Tangy brussels sprout, onions and apple recipes

Brussels Sprouts With Apple

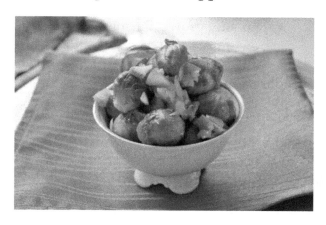

Ingredients *for 4 servings*

- stk Apple
- 500 G Brussels sprouts
- 1 prize salt
- EL Sunflower oil
- stk onions

Preparation

1   Wash and clean the Brussels sprouts. Mince the onions and let them turn glassy in oil.
2   Add water and add the Brussels sprouts. Make the whole thing simmer and add salt.
3   Peel and chop the apples and, after about 10 minutes cooking time, add the Brussels sprouts.

Easy roasted vegetables Recipes

Roasted vegetables with pomegranate

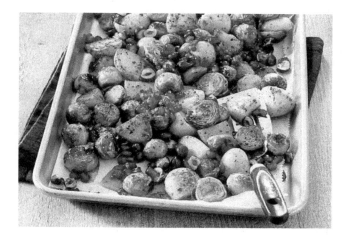

Ingredients *For 4 people*

- 800 g of small potatoes (triplets)
- 600 g Brussels sprouts

- tablespoons olive oil
- 1 teaspoon pepper flakes
- 1 teaspoon coarse sea salt
- pepper
- pomegranate (about 450 g)
- 75 g hazelnut kernels
- tablespoons of maple syrup

Preparation

1 Thoroughly wash the potatoes, grate them dry and halve, or quarter them. Brush, wash and halve Brussels sprouts. Mix potatoes and Brussels sprouts with oil, chili, salt and pepper in a bowl. Distribute the vegetables on a baking tray and roast in the preheated oven (electric cooker: 225 ° C / circulating air: 200 ° C / gas: see manufacturer) for approx. 25 minutes. Turn around once after about 15 minutes.

2 In the meantime halve the pomegranate and tap out the seeds with the help of a spoonful. Chop nuts roughly and add about 10 minutes before the end of the cooking time to the vegetables with maple syrup. Remove vegetables from the oven and sprinkle with pomegranate seeds.

Burst cherry tomatoes with garlic

Cherry Tomato Sauce

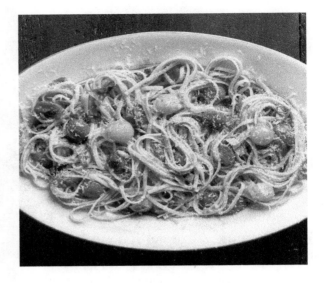

Ingredients

- 1 pound pasta
- Kosher salt
- 1/2 cup olive oil
- large garlic cloves, finely chopped
- pints cherry tomatoes
- 1/2 teaspoon freshly ground black pepper
- Pinch of sugar
- 1 cup coarsely chopped fresh basil
- Freshly grated Parmesan (for serving)

Preparation

1 Cook pasta in a large pot of boiling salted water, stirring occasionally, until al dente; drain and transfer to a large bowl.

2   Meanwhile, heat oil in a 12" skillet or wide heavy saucepan over medium-high. Add garlic, then tomatoes, pepper, sugar, and 1 tsp. salt. Cook, stirring occasionally, until tomatoes burst and release their juices to form a sauce, 6–8 minutes.

3   Toss pasta with tomato sauce and basil. Top with Parmesan.

Hummus-stuffed mini peppers Recipes

Simply barbecue: mini-peppers

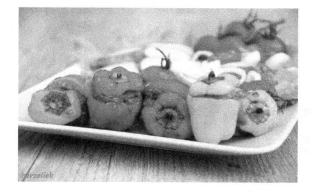

Ingredients

- 500 g ground beef
- 1 onion
- - 3 sprigs of thyme
- 1/2 cup of sour cream
- tablespoons of breadcrumbs
- 1-2 teaspoons salt
- pepper

Preparation

1   Finely chop the onion and the thyme and mix with the sour cream, salt and pepper under the minced meat. Add a little bit of breadcrumbs until the mass does not feel too moist.

2   Now you wash the peppers thoroughly, cut off the lid and remove the seeds. All you have to do is stuff the minced meat into the mini peppers and place them on the grill in a grill bowl.

3   Do not turn the peppers too fast and not too often, they may like to get a little brown, after all, the "roast aroma" is special in this dish.

Baked Zucchini fries recipes

Baked zucchini shells

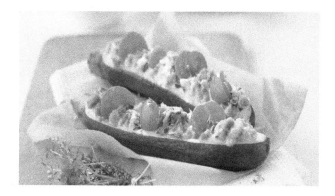

Ingredients

- small zucchini (à ca. 150 g)

- 2-3 spring onions
- fine sausages (approx. 100 g each)
- tablespoons butter
- Salt pepper
- some nutmeg
- 500 ml of vegetable stock
- Fat for the mold
- 125 g cherry tomatoes
- 70 g double-cream cheese
- 2-3 thyme branches

Preparation

1. Clean the zucchini and halve lengthwise. Carefully remove the inside with a spoon and chop. Clean the spring onions and cut into rings.
2. Sauté sausage from the sausages. Sauté with courgette heart and spring onions in hot butter, season with salt, pepper and nutmeg and allow to cool slightly.
3. Pre-heat the courgette halves in boiling broth for 3-5 minutes, drain. Place next to each other in a greased casserole dish. Wash cherry tomatoes and cut in half.
4. Pull cream cheese under the onion sausage mixture and season to taste, then add to the courgette halves. Press in the tomato halves.

Remove thyme leaves from 1 branch, sprinkle over them.
5. Cook the courgette fish in a hot oven at 175 ° C for 30 minutes. Garnish with the remaining thyme.

Soups & Stews

bone broth

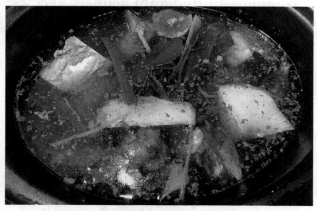

ingredients
2 kg Bovine bone (sand and marrow bones, mixed)
4 Onion (n)
6 liters Water, cold
4 tbsp Apple Cider Vinegar
2 cm ginger root
4 bay leaves

preparation
Halve the onions and roast them together with the bones without adding fat in a large pot until everything has a nice dark color. Meanwhile, peel and quarter the ginger. Pour the bones in cold water, add the ginger, vinegar, bay leaves and allspice and bring to a boil. Adjust the stove so that the liquid stays at the boiling point. Allow to infuse for 18 - 24 hours. If you have the time, you can plan more, because only after 48 hours, all substances should be released from the bones.

Peel or clean the soup vegetables, chop them roughly and add them in the last two hours, then the vegetables should have given their complete taste. If it cooks longer, it could also taste bitter. The vinegar not only provides a round taste, but also serves to ensure that the ingredients are better able to dissolve out of the bones.

After the whole cooking time pour the soup through a sieve, dispose of bones and vegetables. Leave the broth a little and pour it over so gently that the (dirt collected on the bottom) "dirt" remains. Salt as desired.

This is the basic recipe. The broth can be drunk pure, expanded with meat and / or vegetables at will and serves as a strong base for many soups or sauces.

Ramen Base Broth:

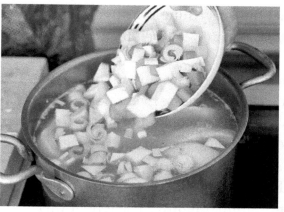

500 g Pork loin or pork loin
100 ml soy sauce
500 g Ramen noodles
4 toe / n garlic
3 Spring onions)
4 Carrot (n)
100 g bean sprouts
4 Egg (s)
1 pinch pepper
1 port. salt
1 tbsp sugar
4 Shiitake mushroom (s) or mushrooms
1 teaspoon Chilli flakes, at will
600 ml vegetable stock

preparation
The broth:
Put the soup chicken with a leek stick, an onion, three to four cloves of garlic, five centimeters of ginger in a piece, pinch of salt, three to four carrots and a handful of algae (optional) in cold water. Add so much water that the chicken is

completely covered. (Choose a pot size that fits everything plus two to three liters of water - a five liter pot is pretty good.)

Slowly bring to a simmer and simmer for at least 3 - 4 hours. Even more delicious is the broth at cooking times of 6 - 8 hours. Should foam arise you can skim this, but you do not have to.

The broth should not cook too much - only simmer lightly. The longer this broth cooks, the better. Then sift the broth. I do not continue using the cooked parts. It is worth to use a good and above all genuine soup chicken, not chicken.

The loin:

Sauté the pork loin in a pan briefly from all sides until it is slightly brownish. Do not fry for too long - only lightly brown! Then put in a pot and add 100 ml of soy sauce (I use Kikkoman because it is naturally brewed) and 50 to 100 ml of rice wine (I use Chinese rice wine). Add 1 tablespoon of sugar, a sliced spring onion (with the green and just a little of the onion) and 3 cm of grated fresh ginger. Add a little water so that the loin is almost completely covered with liquid. Then bring the liquid to a simmer. Again, just simmer gently.

After 40 minutes, remove the loin from the liquid and set aside. The loin before it comes into the soup, cut into approximately 2 - 3 mm thick slices. The loin should come from a good butcher - there are amazing quality differences. A good sirloin is very tender and juicy after this procedure and not tough and dry.

The eggs:

cook and peel four eggs hard. Add the eggs to the loin stock and simmer for 10 minutes. Turn over and over so that they are evenly browned by the brew. When finished, halve and set aside.

The noodles:

You can make your own noodles while the broths are cooking or use Chinese vermicelli from Asiashop. I've had pretty good experiences with Quick-Noodles, but even spaghetti in it tastes very good. If you have a well-stocked shop, you may even get ramen noodles or fresh ramen noodles. The soup:

Cook the noodles but always strictly according to instructions and rather too hard than too soft. When the chicken broth is ready, place it together with the loin stock in a saucepan and season with a few tablespoons of soy sauce and another small shot of rice wine. Maybe even salting, but actually the soy sauce would have to provide enough salt. Then bring everything to a boil again. You can also add water, depending on how strong or diluted you want to have the soup. I leave the broth pure without adding water. When the soup is cooking, all other ingredients should be ready for the next step, especially the noodles. The garnish:

Brew the bean sprouts with hot water in a strainer. Cut the green of two spring onions into rings. Cut out of the Norib leaves small strips (about 2 x 3 cm).

The finish:

Put the soup in a bowl and add so many noodles that the noodles reach just below the surface.

Place two to three slices of loin. The loin can still be sprinkled with coarse pepper.

Place half an egg with the yolk on the edge of the bowl.

Sprinkle a small handful of sprouts and spring onions over it and then put the nori leaf.

Enjoy the sight of the soup, preferably with chopsticks and sipping the broth - then it tastes best. Recipe:

GREEN MISO SOUP

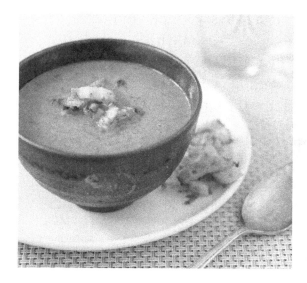

INGREDIENTS:

(gives: 4 servings)

2 tablespoons of grapeseed oil (or another neutral-tasting oil)

1 cup of finely chopped onions

4 cups vegetable stock or water

4 cups of chopped chard leaves (cut stems and leaf ribs first and set aside)

3 heaped tablespoons white or yellow miso paste

1 cup of chopped chard stalks and leaf ribs

2 tbsp breadcrumbs

PREPARATION:

1. Heat half of the oil at medium temperature in a saucepan. Fry the onions softly. Pour in the stock and heat until tender. Then add the chard leaves and cook for 3 minutes. Remove the pot from the heat, stir in the miso and finely puree the soup (if necessary in portions).

2. Heat the remaining oil in a small pan. Fry chard stalks and leaf ribs with the breadcrumbs in it for 1-2 minutes, stirring constantly, until the mixture becomes crispy.

3. Arrange the soup in preheated bowls and garnish with the crunchy mixture.

QUINOA MINESTRONE

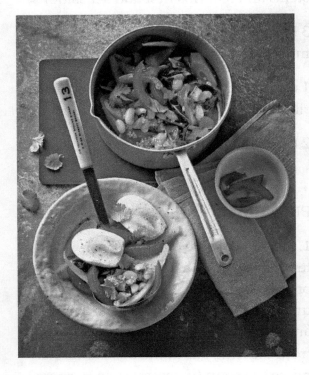

1 onion

1 clove of garlic

250 g of tomatoes

150 g of young zucchini

1 small carrot

100 g of celery

2 stems sage

2 tbsp olive oil

Sea or crystal salt

pepper

600 ml vegetable broth

60g quinoa

½ bunch of parsley

grated peel of ½ organic lemon

50 g freshly grated Parmesan

Peel and dice the onion and clove of garlic. The tomatoes scald, quench, skin and chop. Wash the zucchini, clean, halve lengthwise and slice. Peel the carrot, wash and clean the celery, cut both into slices. Wash, pluck and chop the sage leaves.

Heat the oil in a pot. Fry the onion and garlic in a glassy sauce. Add the vegetables, season with sage, salt and pepper. Add the broth, bring to the boil and sprinkle with the quinoa. Cover and cook for 15-20 minutes on a low heat.

Meanwhile, wash the parsley, shake it dry, pluck the leaves and chop. Mix with the lemon peel. Season the soup with salt and pepper, sprinkle with the parsley mixture and the Parmesan cheese on top.

Tip for the office: Fill the hot soup in a preheated thermo container, seal well - and enjoy lunch.

Chop the onion, celery and leek and cook with the broccoli and spices in the beef broth for 20 minutes.

Add the melted cheese, let it melt for a short time and then puree it.

Spicy broccoli soup

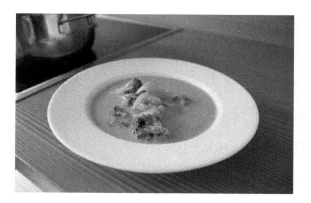

ingredients

1 Broccoli, fresh

1 Onion (n)

1 kl. Disk (s) Celery, fresh

1 pole / s leek

100 g cream cheese

½ TL Chilli flakes, dried

1 pinch Pepper, black, freshly ground

1 tbsp Parsley, dried

1 liter beef broth

preparation

Creamy tomato soup

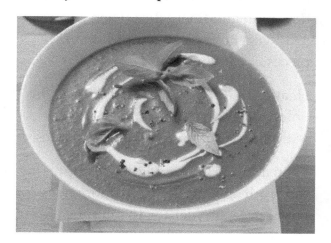

Ingredients

1 stk onion

1 Federation Suppengrün

1 EL oil

1 TL marjoram

1 TL Flour

0.5 l vegetable stock

1 can Tomatoes, peeled

1 prize salt

1 prize pepper

1 prize sugar

100 G whipped cream

preparation

For the creamy tomato soup, first remove the onion and finely dice. Then clean the soup vegetables and cut into small pieces.

Heat the oil in a saucepan and sauté the onion cubes and the soup vegetables with the marjoram for about 5 minutes.

Then add the flour and then with stirring the broth and stir the peeled tomatoes with juice - simmer for 15 minutes.

Then finely puree the soup with the blender, stir in the whipped cream and season with salt, pepper and sugar.

Cauliflower soup

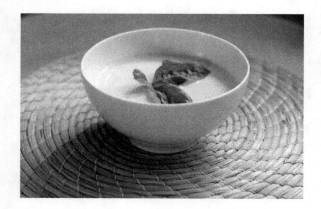

Ingredients: for 4 people

1 medium cauliflower (600 g)

750 ml water

1 level tsp salt

150 ml milk (1,5% fat)

100 ml sweet cream (30% fat)

1 tablespoon flour stock cubes (finished product)

salt

white pepper

Toasted bread cubes:

4 slices Toasted bread

1 heaped tsp butter (15 g)

parsley to sprinkle

Picture of cauliflower soup

Click on picture to enlarge

Preparation:

For the cauliflower soup recipe, first clean the cauliflower, cut into florets, wash and strain in a sieve.

Put salted water and milk in a saucepan and bring to a boil.

You should not lose sight of the pot, as the milk overcooks too much heat.

Put the cauliflower florets into the boiling liquid, bring to the boil again, then slowly boil the cauliflower in about 20 minutes.

Remove the pot, blend the cauliflower with the liquid using a hand blender, or squeeze the whole mixture through a strainer.

Mix the flour with the cream in a small bowl, stir into the cauliflower soup, and at the same time add a broth cube to the pan.

Put the pan back onto the hot plate and boil the cauliflower soup thoroughly with a whisk, stirring gently, then cook for about 5 minutes. Now is the moment where you can extend the amount of cauliflower soup, as desired.

If desired, add some more broth or water and thicken with a little extra flour.

Finally, season the cauliflower soup to taste with some salt and white ground pepper.

Sprinkle the cauliflower soup with plenty of fresh parsley, serve.

Roasted bread cubes taste very good with this simple, home-style cauliflower soup.

For the preparation of roasted bread cubes, Cut the toast into small cubes, place in a coated frying pan, without additional fat, and roast the bread cubes round tenderly golden-yellow to light-brown with constant use of a spatula.

Pull the pan aside and only then add 1 heaped tsp butter to the pan and turn the still hot croutons into it.

In this way you get crispy, tasting wonderful butter, relatively low-fat roasted bread cubes.

Serve the bread cubes with the cauliflower soup.

Shchi

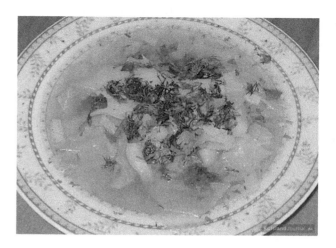

Ingredients

2 l water

200 g Soupmeat

750 g (or a small head) white cabbage

3 onions

1 big each Carrot and tomato (or 1 tbsp tomato paste)

2 potatoes

1 teaspoon Caraway seed

2 bay leaves

10 black peppercorns

4 Garlic cloves

2 tablespoons each Parsley and dill

200 g sour cream

Salt pepper

Put the meat on little water (enough to cover the meat), heat it up and bring it to a boil until it forms foam. Pour away the water and remove the foam residue from the pot. Refill the meat with hot water, bring to the boil, add a whole onion, 2 cloves of garlic and bay leaves and cook over low heat for about 2 hours.

Throw away the cooked onion and bay leaves from the broth. Remove meat and cut it to size.

Shchi preparation

Remove white cabbage from outer leaves, cut out the stump. Grate cabbage.

Finely dice the remaining 2 onions and garlic. Cut the potato into fine strips. Grate carrot.

Put everything together with the white cabbage in the boiling meat broth (or boiling water) and cook on low heat for 15 minutes.

Wash tomato, cut into quarters and add to the soup with peppercorns and cumin. Simmer for another 10 minutes.

When the meat has been removed from the broth, it will also come into the pot about 5 minutes before the end of cooking.

Season the cabbage soup with salt and pepper.

Sprinkle shchi with plenty of parsley and dill and serve with plenty of sour cream (about 2 tablespoons each).

Fast Red Lentil Dal

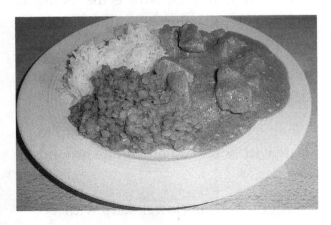

ingredients

1 Onion (s), diced

1 Garlic clove (s), chopped

1 tbsp Ginger, chopped

something oil

3 cups / n Lentils, red

something yogurt

something coriander leaves

something Onion (s), (onion rings)

½ TL salt

1 teaspoon, heaped turmeric

1 ½ tsp curry powder

½ TL Spice mixture, (Garam Masala)

preparation

Heat some oil in a saucepan, sauté onions, garlic and ginger. Then add all the spices except salt and roast, stir well so it does not matter. Now come the lenses. I take coffee cups, not pots. Mix everything, add approx. 250 ml of water and simmer for approx. 15 minutes until the lentils are soft, but not mushy, if necessary. Add some more water. Season with salt until finally.

On the plates, Then make yoghurt, freshly chopped cilantro and a few onion rings in one go.

BUTTERNUT CREAM SOUP WITH COCONUT MILK

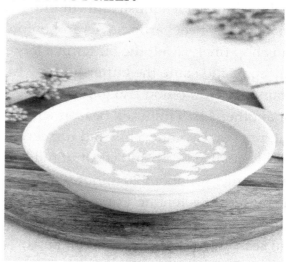

INGREDIENTS

- 1200 g of butternut squash

- 2 garlic cloves

- 2 onions

- 1 tablespoon butter

- salt + freshly ground pepper

- about 1/2 teaspoon cayenne pepper

- some chili from the mill* or a few chilli flakes

- 2 tsp turmeric

- 700 ml vegetable broth

- 800 ml coconut milk

- 1 tbsp lemon juice

- fresh coriander or fresh parsley to taste

PREPARATION:

Peel the butternut squash and cut into small pieces. Peel garlic cloves and onion and chop finely. Melt the butter in a large saucepan and sauté the butternut for 2 to 3 minutes. Add onion and garlic and fry for another 4 to 5 minutes. Season with salt, pepper, cayenne, chili and turmeric. Add vegetable broth and coconut milk and simmer for about 20 minutes until the butternut is tender. Puree the butternut cream soup with the blender and season with lemon juice, salt and pepper. Wash coriander or parsley, shake dry and chop, if necessary. Serve with the butternut cream soup.

Vegetable soup with herbal turkey balls

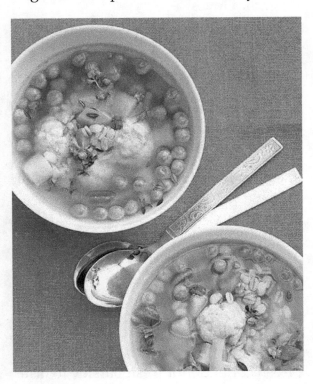

Ingredients:

• 400 g turkey breast;

• 2 potatoes;

• 1 onion;

• 1 carrot;

• 200 g of cauliflower;

• 170 g of frozen green peas;

• ½ small bunch of parsley;

• 1, 5 liters. water

• 2 TBSP. l small pasta;

• 2 TBSP. l sunflower oil;

• 1 tsp salts;

• ¼ tsp. black pepper

Cook

1. Wash the cauliflower and divide it into small twigs. Chop the onion, dice the potatoes and grate the carrot. Wash parsley and chop.

2. Pour oil into a deep pan and heat it. Add the onion to the hot oil and lower slightly, then add the carrot, mix and fry until the ingredients are tender.

3. Put the potato cubes in a saucepan, add water, place on the heat, bring to a boil and cook.

4. Wash turkey breast, chop, season with salt and pepper, sprinkle with parsley and mix well. From the cooked filling with wet hands form small meatballs.

5. Add all the meatballs to the boiling soup one at a time and stir gently with a spoon so that nothing sticks together. Season the salted soup and cook for 3-4 minutes.

6. After this time, add cauliflower twigs and frozen peas to the soup and cook for 5 minutes. Then lay out the onion with the carrot and boil for another 5 minutes.

7. At the end of cooking, add the pasta and, if necessary, add salt (universal seasoning). Boil the soup for a few minutes, remove from the heat, cover and leave to rest for about 20 minutes.

8. After 20 minutes put the soup with turkey meatballs in a plate and serve with bread, vegetables and vegetables.

Avocado Chicken Soup

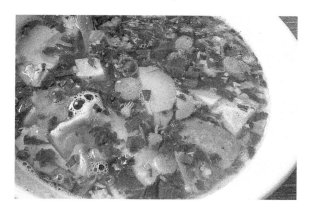

ingredients

300 g Chicken breast

1 Avocado (s)

2 Spring onions)

1 handful coriander leaves

700 ml broth

1 toe garlic

1 Lime (n)

something oil

salt and pepper

preparation

Heat the oil (if you like it a bit more hot, take chilli oil) in a saucepan, lightly salt the chicken breast and fry gently all around. Once it's through, take out of the pot.

Now cut the spring onions into fine rings and add to the hot oil, sauté briefly, then squeeze the garlic.

Shortly before the garlic begins to brown, deglaze with the broth.

Now tear the chicken breast into the smallest possible pieces and put it back into the soup. Squeeze out the lime and add the juice to the soup.

Remove the avocado from the skin and cut into pieces that are not too small, divide them on two large soup bowls, season with salt and pepper, add the hot

soup and sprinkle with coarsely chopped
coriander leaves.

CHAPTER 2

5 Kitchen Staples That Everyone Should Have

Every healthy kitchen should always have these important things at hand.

1. nutritional yeast

It may seem intimidating at first, but it's nothing to be afraid of! This inactivated yeast is a powerhouse of nutrients that provides a great source of protein, B vitamins, folic acid, zinc, iron, magnesium, and the list goes on. It has a savory, nutty, cheesy taste and tastes great with salads, popcorn, vegetables, pasta, and soups.

2. Raw almond butter

Almond butter can help lower cholesterol, keep you full for longer, control blood sugar, and support weight loss (despite healthy fats!).

3. Chia seeds

These magical seeds work wonders in the body. Soaked in liquid, they take up nine times their weight, which means they form a jelly-like texture. These energizing seeds have twice as much protein as all other seeds, five times as much calcium as milk, twice as much potassium as bananas, three times as much iron as spinach, and a large amount of heart-healthy omega-3 and omega-6 fatty acids. Mix these seeds in your morning smoothie or make a delicious chia seed pudding!

4. Lenses

Lentils make a filling lunch or dinner and have an unlimited shelf life. Lentils are high in fiber, iron, B vitamins, and protein. The combinations are endless: lentil soup, lentil salad, lentil burger, lentil curry.

5. sea vegetables

This is the same kelp used for sushi. It has been found that Nori significantly reduces breast cancer risk and cholesterol levels. Not only is Nori used for sushi, but it is also great for making salad wraps, vegetable buns, or seaweed salad!

Hazelnut And Almond Macaroons

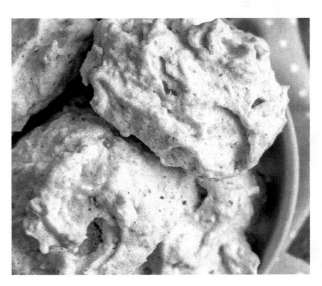

- 140 g protein (from about 4 eggs size M)

- 60 g of granulated sugar
- 130 g of powdered sugar
- 90 g of chopped hazelnuts
- 90 g of ground almonds
- 40 g almond flakes
- 1 pinch of cinnamon
- 1 pinch of salt
- Mark a vanilla pod

Roast the almond flakes lightly in a frying pan without fat and allow to cool. Put chopped hazelnuts, almonds, ground almonds, cinnamon and vanilla in a small bowl and sift the icing sugar. Preheat the oven to 145 ° C (top and bottom heat).

Beat the egg whites in a clean mixing bowl first on a medium, then on the fastest stage until frothy but not yet stiff. Add salt and granulated sugar, then beat until stiff. The egg whites should shine and stand on the turned whisk in firm tips upwards.

Carefully lift the powdered sugar and nut mixture in three portions with a spatula under the egg whites. Place the mass on a grid covered with baking paper with the help of two tablespoons and bake on the middle rack for 40-45 minutes. Allow the macaroons to cool, then carefully remove from the baking paper and store in a tight metal box.

Lemon dressing

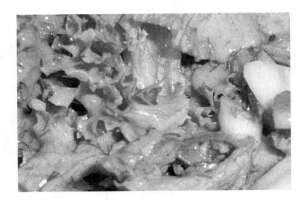

ingredients For

- 6 tbsp lemon juice
- 1 tbsp Lemon (s) - Peel, finely sieved
- 1 tbsp Mustard (Dijonsenf)
- 1 tbsp sugar
- 200 ml Olive oil, (not extra virgin)
- salt and pepper

preparation

Mix the lemon juice, peel, mustard, sugar, salt and pepper with the whisk, then slowly add the oil while stirring until the dressing has a creamy consistency. Goes well with crustaceans, fish, vegetables and fine lettuce.

Paleo Caesar Dressing

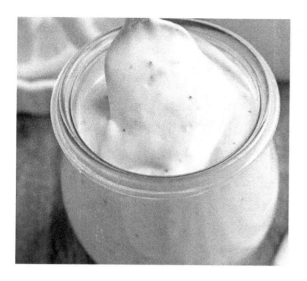

Aioli

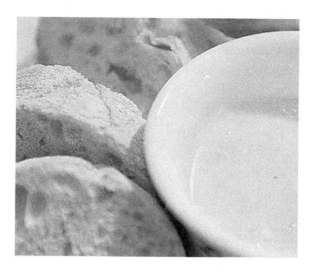

INGREDIENTS

- 2 eggs room temperature
- 1 ounce anchovies 1/2 can or about 5 filets
- 2 cloves garlic*
- 1/2 teaspoon salt
- 1/2 teaspoon pepper
- 1 tablespoon coconut vinegar or apple cider vinegar
- Juice of 1 lemon
- 2 - 2 1/2 cups light olive oil

INSTRUCTIONS

In a large mouth mason jar, combine eggs, anchovies, garlic, salt, pepper, vinegar, and lemon juice. Using an immersion blender, blend until completely smooth. About 30 seconds.

With the blender on, slowly pour in olive oil and move blender up and down in the jar until all oil is added and mixture is thick.

ingredients For

- 3 toe / n garlic
- egg yolk
- 250 ml Oil, neutral (eg sunflower oil)
- 1 teaspoon lemon juice
- salt and pepper

preparation

Place warm egg yolk in a bowl.

Peel garlic and process into a mortar in a mortar. Always add salt to make the paste bind. Then mix in a bowl with the egg yolk and a dash of lemon juice.

Add oil slowly, first drop by drop, later in a thin stream, whipping vigorously with the whisk all the while.

Be careful, add the oil too fast, the mass will clot, ie the process of splashing will take time!

Finally, season again and, if necessary, season with salt and pepper.

Juicy apricot and redcurrant slices with pistachio pesto

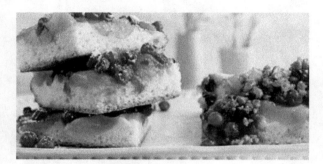

ingredients

- 1 kg of ripe apricots
- 500 g of redcurrants
- a little + 75 g soft butter
- 450 g + some flour
- 1 packet of baking soda
- 125 g + 1 tbsp sugar
- 1 packet of vanilla sugar
- salt
- 100 ml of milk
- 100 ml of oil
- egg (size M)
- 250 g of low-fat quark
- organic lime
- 100 g pistachios
- powdered sugar

preparation

Wash apricots, halve, stone and cut into wide slices. Carefully wash currants and brush with a fork from the panicles. A fat pan (deep baking sheet, about 32 x 39 cm) grease well.

Preheat oven (electric cooker: 200 ° C / circulating air: 175 ° C / gas: see manufacturer).

For the dough mix 450 g of flour, baking powder, 125 g of sugar, vanilla sugar and 1 pinch of salt. Add milk, oil, egg and quark and knead with the dough hooks of the mixer. Roll out the curd oil dough on the drip pan.

Press edges and corners with floured hands.

Spread 75 g butter in little flakes on the pastry. Give apricots and redcurrants. Bake cake in hot oven for 30-35 minutes. Remove and allow to cool on a wire rack.

For the pesto wash lime hot, pat dry and rub the skin. Squeeze out lime. Chop pistachios, lime zest and 1 tbsp sugar in a universal shredder or chop with a large kitchen knife.

Stir in the juice. Cut cake into pieces, dust with powdered sugar. To give the pistachio pesto.

Romesco sauce

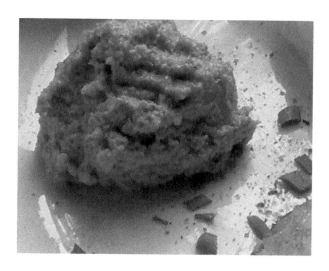

ingredients

- 4 pcs of sun-ripened tomatoes
- 50 gr. Hazelnuts without skin
- 50 gr. Almonds without skin
- 4 garlic cloves
- 30 ml 30 ml olive oil cold pressed
- 3 tablespoons tomato juice
- 4 St. 4 chilis fresh & amp; quot; ancho & amp; amp; quot; and red
- 2 pieces of sliced toasted bread or breadcrumbs
- 1 tbsp red wine vinegar
- 1 tbsp red wine, dry and fruity
- 1 Msp. 1 Msp. Sea salt or to taste
- 1 Msp. Pimenton de la Vera or Paprika Rosenscharf
- 1 pc paprika red fresh

preparation

Remove the tomatoes from the stalk and slice.

Free the peppers from stalk and inner life and cut strips 2 cm.

Put the tomatoes and peppers in the preheated oven and lightly toast for 1 hour at 150 ° C on baking paper, or better dry them so that the aroma and sweetness are better for the sauce. In the middle of the process, after half an hour, put the garlic cloves with the skin and roast.

Lightly toast the almonds and hazelnuts in a pan to enhance the aroma. Also goes in the oven but be careful not to burn them, go quickly.

Put the cooled paprika and tomatoes in a blender, remove the garlic from the skin and add to the tomato / pepper. Add the almonds and hazelnuts.

Then mix everything to a fine paste, mix the tomato juice, add the chilies cleaned and freed from the seeds.

The white bread with mix, the red wine vinegar and the olive oil, the red wine at the end of the sauce should be too thick with red wine or with oil to produce the desired consistency to taste.

Easy pasta pot with white beans

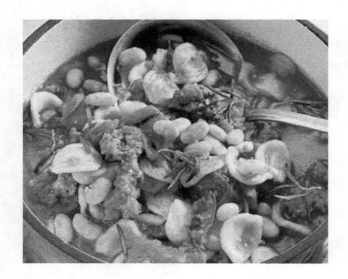

something. Pour 1 1/4 l of water, boil, stir in broth. Season with pepper and 1 tsp paprika. Add the pasta and simmer for about 18 minutes, stirring occasionally.

Rinse beans, drain. Heat in the last 2 minutes. Season with salt and pepper.

ingredients

- onion
- cloves of garlic
- branch rosemary
- 2 tbsp olive oil
- 300 g pig fat
- 1 tin (s) (à 850 ml) tomatoes
- 2 tablespoons vegetable broth (instant)
- pepper
- Sweet paprika
- salt
- 250 g small pasta (eg orecchiette)
- 1 tin (s) (à 425 ml) white bean seeds

preparation

Peel and dice the onion and garlic. Wash the rosemary, remove the needles.

Heat oil in a large saucepan. Roast Mett crumbly in it. Fry the onion, garlic and rosemary briefly. Add tomatoes, mince

Chapter 3:

mango turmeric lassi

ingredients

1 mango (about 350 g)

200 g skyr

2 Msp. Ground turmeric

2 tablespoons of agave syrup

1 tbsp lime juice

3 ice cubes (as you like)

preparation

Peel mango, cut into slices from the stone and roughly cut into pieces.

Together with skyr, 100 ml of water, turmeric, agave syrup, lime juice and if you want with ice cubes in a powerful blender to puree.

Would you like it more fluid? Mix another 1-2 tablespoons of water under the lassi.

Sweet fig smoothie

ingredients

2 cups of spinach fresh

5-10 raspberry leaves

1/2 avocado

1 cup of mixed fresh berries e.g. Raspberries, blueberries, redcurrants, blackberries

3 figs fresh

1 mango ripe

Juice of 2 oranges

instructions

Clean ingredients and cut to the size of the mix.

Halve the avocado, core it and remove the pulp!

Do everything in the blender and mix until smooth consistency!

Enjoy a fig smoothie from the heart!

Matcha berry smoothie

250 ml pear juice

125 g mixed berries

1 tsp honey

1 tbsp oatmeal

½ teaspoon matcha tea

That's how it's done:

Pear juice, mixed berries, honey, oatmeal and Matcha tea in the blender, mix well.

Ready is your smoothie!

Pumpkin Pie Smoothie

ingredients

135 g (½ cup) pumpkin from the tin

240 ml (1 cup) of milk

80 ml (⅓ cup) sweetened condensed milk

1 tablespoon of vanilla yogurt

1 teaspoon of pumpkin pie spice mixture

130 g (1 cup) ice cube

preparation

Put all ingredients into the Vitamix container in the order listed and seal with the lid.

Select setting 1.

Switch on the device, gradually increase the speed to level 10 and then up to "high".

Mix for 45 seconds or to the desired consistency.

Serve with whipped cream and a touch of cinnamon.

CARROTS PINEAPPLE GINGER SMOOTHIE

INGREDIENTS

3 carrots

15gr ginger

½ pineapple

1 banana

1 ½ limes

100ml of water

PREPARATION

So that the carrots can be mixed, you first peel the carrots. Then you throw them in a pot with a ground cover water, so they do not fry. Now they are cooked so that the carrots soften.

In the meantime you can halve the pineapple and cut out the pulp. Then you give the pineapple with the peeled banana and the juice of limes in the blender. You weigh the ginger and peel it. Give this with the now soft carrots together in the blender.

Now add some water and mix everything properly.

Apricot Cherry Tart with Frangipane:

For the dough:

60 g flour

60 g powdered sugar

2 tbsp powdered sugar

1/4 tsp salt

170 g cold butter, cut into small cubes

For the Frangipane:

65 g sugar

65 g soft butter

1 egg (size M)

100 g finely ground almonds

Scattered peel of 1 organic lemon

3 tablespoons milk or whipped cream

2 teaspoons flour

10-12 apricots, each cut in 6 columns

25-30 cherries, gutted and halved

Knead all ingredients together well for the dough and refrigerate for 1 hour in the fridge.

Preheat the oven to 190 ° C top and bottom heat.

For the Frangipane filling, stir the soft butter and the sugar until creamy. Then stir in the egg. Stir in the ground almonds, then the citrus peel and finally the milk or cream. Then stir in the flour briefly and quickly.

Press the dough into a greased Tart mold. Then fill in the Frangipane. Cover with apricot slices and cherry halves.

Bake the tart for about 35 minutes until the dough is golden brown. Remove and allow to cool.

apple spritzer

ingredients For

300 ml apple juice

1 splash Lemon juice, freshly squeezed

1 Cinnamon sticks)

Possibly. Sugar, brown, optional

preparation

Fill the apple spritzer with the lemon juice in a large glass. Put the cinnamon stick in the liquid, put the glass in the microwave. Heat at 800 watts for 2 minutes and 20 seconds.

Migas with Black Beans

INGREDIENTS

Crispy tortilla strips

4 small corn tortillas

1 ½ teaspoons olive oil

Salt

Spicy black beans (half of these peppers go into the eggs)

1 small red onion, chopped

1 red bell pepper, seeded and chopped

1 poblano pepper or 1 additional bell pepper, seeded and chopped

1 jalapeño pepper, seeded and chopped

4 garlic cloves, pressed or minced

2 teaspoons olive oil

1 teaspoon ground cumin

1 (15 ounce) can of black beans, drained

3 tablespoons water

Squeeze of lime juice or splash of sherry vinegar

Scrambled eggs

8 eggs

3 tablespoons cream or milk of choice

¼ teaspoon salt

Freshly ground black pepper

2 teaspoons olive oil

½ to ¾ cup grated Monterey Jack cheese or cheddar cheese

Garnishes

Chopped cilantro

Salsa and/or hot sauce of choice

More tortillas, warmed (optional)

Diced avocado (optional)

INSTRUCTIONS

Preheat oven to 425 degrees Fahrenheit and line a baking sheet with parchment paper while you're at it. Scramble 8 eggs with 3 tablespoons cream/milk, ¼

teaspoon salt and a few twists of freshly ground black pepper. Set the eggs aside for later.

Slice 4 tortillas into short, thin strips (see photos). Transfer the strips to your prepared baking sheet, then toss with 1 ½ teaspoons olive oil until lightly and evenly coated. Arrange them in a single layer and sprinkle with salt. Bake until crispy, flipping halfway, about 8 to 10 minutes.

Meanwhile, cook the pepper-and-onion mixture. In a medium saucepan over medium heat, warm 2 teaspoons olive oil. Add the chopped onion, bell pepper, jalapeño, garlic and a dash of salt. Cook, stirring often, until the onions are turning translucent and the peppers are tender, about 5 minutes. Transfer half of the mixture to a bowl for later and return the pot to heat.

To the pot, add 1 teaspoon ground cumin and sauté until fragrant, stirring constantly, about 30 seconds. Add the drained black beans and 3 tablespoons water. Stir to combine. Reduce heat to low, cover and simmer until you're ready to serve.

Once you have your crispy tortilla strips and reserved pepper mixture ready, you can scramble the eggs. In a 10-inch non-stick or well-seasoned cast iron skillet, warm 2 teaspoons olive oil over medium heat. Swirl the pan so it's evenly coated with oil. Add the peppers from your bowl to the skillet, then whisk your egg mixture one last time and pour it into the skillet.

Scramble the eggs by pushing the mixture around and 'round and 'round until they're about three-fourths set. Fold in the crispy tortilla strips and cheese and continue cooking until the eggs are scrambled to your liking. Remove from heat.

Remove the beans from heat. Use a fork to mash up about half the beans, then stir in a squeeze of lime or splash of vinegar. Season to taste with salt and pepper.

Divide migas and black beans into individual serving bowls/plates. Top with a sprinkle of chopped cilantro. Serve with salsa, warmed tortillas (optional) and diced avocado (optional) on the side.

Spinach and leek frittata

ingredients

spinach

250 g , spinach leaves (fresh or frozen)

Leek

1 pole (s), large , in thin strips

Chicken egg /

6 pieces

food starch

2 tsp

Milk, low fat, 1.5% fat

100 ml

Parmesan / Montello Parmesan

1 tbsp., Grated

sea-salt 1 pinch

pepper 1 pinch

manual

Preheat oven to 180 ° C. Place a baking tin, approx. Ø 20 cm, with parchment paper.

Blanch spinach in boiling water for about 2 minutes; drain and express lightly. Prepare TK spinach according to the package instructions. Chop cooled in rough strips.

Blanch the leek separately in 3 minutes; let drain, also express easily. Distribute both vegetables on the bottom of the baking pan.

Stir eggs, starch, milk and spices together; pour over the vegetables. Press the mass with a fork in the mold.

Spread the cheese over it, bake for about 18-20 minutes until the frittata has risen and is golden-brown.

10 min. allow to cool, remove the mold and serve cut into small pieces of cake.

Fried rice with egg

ingredients

600 g Rice, cooked

3 Egg (s)

½ Lemon (s), juice of it

thyme

Salt or soy sauce

pepper

oil

preparation

Heat pan or wok and let oil in it get hot. Add the cooked rice and stir-fry for a while, keeping it at the highest level. Season with pepper and salt or soy sauce, lemon juice and thyme. Whisk the eggs over and give, stir again really well, so that there are beautiful "Eierfetzchen". Season with pepper and salt or soy sauce.

Stir well after each ingredient, before adding the next one.

The length of the roasting time depends on the desired tan and consistency of the rice and the eggs. I always roast the rice for about 10 minutes, then come first the spices and the egg and then I let it fry as a whole again about 10 minutes.

Of course you can also vegetables (eg peppers or peas) or meat (but that should then make the roast) to give it, but it tastes best, even for breakfast or as a warm addition to the brunch.

Salmon trout on wild garlic puree with fried garlic

INGREDIENTS

Salmon trout fillet

Butter liquid for the wild garlic puree

6 big ones potatoes

Almond milk

salt and pepper

2 tablespoons Wild garlic chopped

plentiful butter

PREPARATION

first boil the potatoes soft - then peel and finely crush together with the almond milk, a little salt and pepper and wild garlic - ALTERNATIVE: my wild garlic comes at this time of year of course from the freezer, who has no wild garlic available, who could also use finely chopped rocket and some finely chopped garlic

Wash the fish, dab dry and remove all bones with tweezers - marinate with a little lemon juice - then brush with a brush lukewarm, liquid butter - brush a heat-resistant mold with the butter, put the fish on it, season with some sea salt and freshly ground pepper - Cook in the preheated oven at 120 degrees for approx. 14 minutes

bisect the garlic bulb in the middle - cut in a dry pan over medium heat while gently toasting the garlic cloves out of the shell ... the garlic gets very mild in the taste and almost a little sweet !!! tastes very fine !!!

Baked apple-Chia Pudding

ingredients

250 ml Soy milk (soy drink), (vanilla), alternatively another vegetable milk

4 tbsp Chia seeds

2 big ones apples

4 tbsp cane sugar

½ TL cinnamon

4 tsp raspberry jam

4 tbsp Walnuts, crushed

preparation

Let the chia seeds swell in the soymilk for at least 4 hours, preferably overnight.

Then make the baked apples. Peel the apples, core them and cut into small pieces. Add cane sugar, ground cinnamon, raspberry jam and crushed walnuts.

Put in the oven for 20 minutes at 200 ° C. Then let the baked apple pieces cool down a bit.

Now the whole thing is done. First, give the chia pudding in Gals. Then arrange the baked apple pieces on it - done.

Breakfast yoghurt with spelled sprouts

ingredients

70 g Sprouts (spelled sprouts, from approx. 40 g spelled grains)

150 g Natural yoghurt (3.8% fat) or natural soy yoghurt

1 tbsp Raisins, soaked

something Water for soaking

1 Msp. vanilla powder

1 m. -Large Apple

preparation

Drain the soaked raisins. Grate the apple with the shell and mix with the other ingredients.

Spelled sprouts are easy to grow from organic spelled grains. Soak the spelled for 12 hours and then germinate for 3 - 4 days. Rinse the germs twice daily. I prefer to use germination glasses for germination.

Spelled sprouts taste slightly sweetish (but not as sweet as wheat sprouts) and have a bit of a bite. In addition, spelled is rich in vitamin B3 (niacin), potassium and magnesium.

Healthy Banana Oatmeal Pancakes

ingredients For

1 cup Oatmeal, tender

1 Banana (s), ripe

1 Egg (s)

60 ml milk

1 teaspoon, heaped ground cinnamon

something Butter for the pan

preparation

Crush the banana to a pulp with a fork or blender. Grind the oatmeal into flour, preferably with a flour mill, if necessary also with a blender.

Put all ingredients in a container. Purée until a smooth dough is formed. Put some butter in a small pan for frying and fry the pancakes in portions golden brown. For each serving, the recipe gives about 2-3 cakes.

As a side dish it tastes wonderful a bit of natural yoghurt with fresh fruit from the season. Optionally, but also with red groats, quark and banana pieces a treat.

CHAPTER FOUR

Snacks and sides recipes

Chinese eggplants

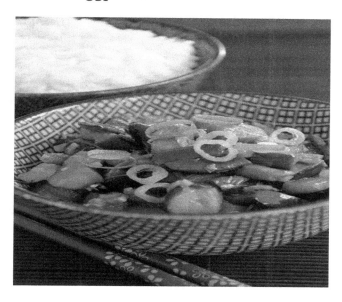

Ingredients *for 2 servings*

- 2 eggplants
- peanut oil or a neutral for frying
- 1-2 cloves of garlic
- 1 piece of thick piece of ginger
- 2 scallions
- 1 tablespoon sambal oelek
- 1 teaspoon sugar
- 2 tablespoons soy sauce
- 1-2 tablespoons rice vinegar
- Sesame oil for seasoning

Preparation

8. Peel the garlic and ginger and chop very finely.

9. Clean the spring onions, cut away the root and the dark, dry green and chop finely.

10. For the sauce, mix soy sauce, sugar, rice vinegar and Sambal Oelek with some sesame oil (for taste).

11. Wash, dry and dice the aubergines and sauté in very hot oil until they have a nice brown color on all sides.

12. Remove from the wok and mix with the sauce.

13. Add the garlic, ginger and spring onions to the remaining oil and fry gently. When a delicious scent develops, add the aubergines and sauce to the wok, mix well and fry for a few minutes.

14. A nice side dish to rice. Or just like that.

Simplest guacamole

Guacamole

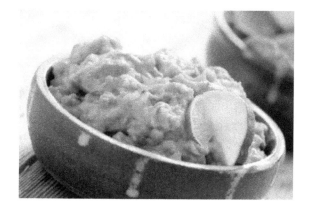

Ingredients *for 16 servings*

- 2 stk mild, red peppers
- 1 stk lime
- 2 stk ripe avocados
- spr Tabasco
- prize salt
- stk tomatoes
- prize Pepper (mill)
- stk small onion
- stk clove of garlic

Preparation

5   For this Mexican guacamole, first cut the peppers in half lengthwise, corer them and finely dice them. Peel the onion and cut into small pieces. Juice lime. Finely chop the tomatoes (it is best to add them to the boiling water, blanch , skin and core).

6   Then halve the avocados, remove the kernel and remove the pulp from the peel with a spoon - cut and slice avocados properly

7   Then puree the avocado meat and the lime juice (or lemon juice) in a blender.

8   Season the avocado puree with salt, pepper and Tabasco. Add the peppercorn cubes, onion pieces and diced tomatoes to the puree and let it steep for 15 minutes.

Spicy two-bean dip recipes

BEAN DIP

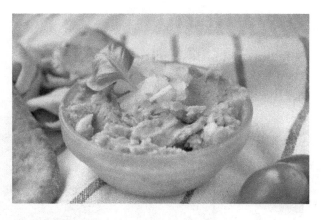

Ingredients *for 2 servings*

- 250G Beans (white)
- stk onion
- stk garlic
- EL butter
- TL tomato paste
- TL paprika
- prize Salt pepper
- shot olive oil

Preparation

4   Put white beans in water overnight or take them out of the can and wash thoroughly. Boil the beans in salted water until they are cooked. The beans are now mashed with a little boiled water.

5   Finely chop the onion and sauté in a pan with a little butter, add the pressed garlic clove, the beans and add the tomato puree. Pour some water if necessary. Turn down the heat.

6   Now season with the finely chopped parsley, salt, pepper, paprika and a dash of olive oil.

Simmer until it thickened nicely. Serve the dip with bread or something else for dipping.

Cashew hummus dip recipes

Cashew Hummus

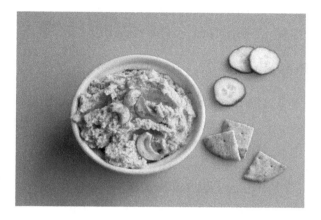

Ingredients

- 1 540-mL can chickpeas , drained and rinsed well
- 1/2 cup roasted, unsalted cashews
- 1/4 cup olive oil
- 1 tbsp fresh lemon juice
- 1/2 tsp finely chopped garlic
- 1/4 tsp ground cumin
- 1/4 tsp salt
- 3-4 tsp water

Preparation

3 Combine chickpeas with cashews, olive oil, lemon juice, garlic, cumin and salt in the bowl of a food processor. Purée until well combined.

4 Scrape down the sides of the bowl and continue blending, adding water gradually until hummus is the texture you like.

Avocado-Apple-prosciutto wrap recipes

Avocado Ham Wraps

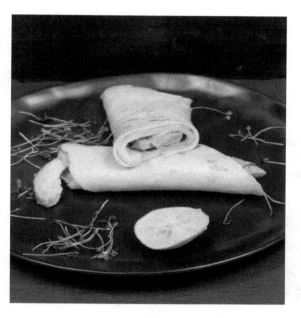

Ingredients

- 11/2 avocado
- slices of cooked ham
- 75 grams of wheat flour
- 25 grams of spelled wholemeal flour
- 1 pinch of salt
- 250 milliliters of milk
- 1 egg
- 1 teaspoon rapeseed oil
- 1 splash of lemon

- Freshly ground pepper

Preparation

4 Peel avocado and cut into slices. Drizzle with lemon juice.
5 Mix a pancake with flour, salt, milk and egg. Heat the oil in a non-stick pan and bake out 3 pancakes.
6 Cover each pancake with 2 slices of cooked ham and half an avocado. Peppers and then roll into a wrap. Cut to serve in the middle.

Roasted chickpeas Recipes

Roasted chickpeas

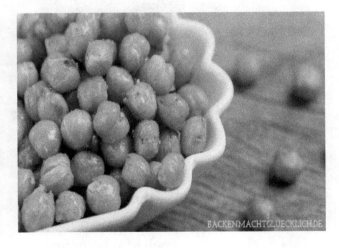

Ingredients

- cans of pre-cooked chickpeas per 250g drained weight; alternatively approx. 200g raw
- tablespoons of olive oil
- 1.5 tablespoons of sea salt
- 2 teaspoons paprika powder
- 1 pinch of chilli powder
- 1 pinch of garlic powder

Preparation

5 Drain the chickpeas from the tin, rinse and then dry or dab well. (Raw chickpeas must first be soaked overnight and then cooked for about 1.5 hours.) Preheat the oven to 190 degrees top and bottom heat. Cover a tin with baking paper.
6 Mix the dry chickpeas in a bowl with the olive oil. Spread on the plate and bake for about 25 minutes (depending on how crispy you want it or how your stove heats).
7 Twist or shake twice during the baking time to make the chickpeas brown evenly. Watch at the end of the baking time so they do not get too dark.
8 Remove from the oven, still hot with salt and spices and warm.

Salt & Vinegar Chips

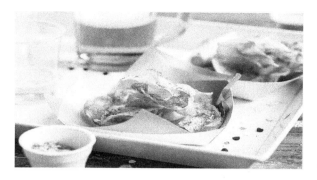

Ingredients for *2 servings*

- gold potatoes
- cups vinegar (480 mL)
- 1 tablespoon salt
- 1 tablespoon pepper

Preparation

8 Carefully slice 3 gold potatoes into ⅛ inch (3 mm) slices using a knife or mandoline.
9 In a large bowl, coat chips with vinegar so all are submerged, allow to sit for 30 minutes (the longer they sit the more vinegary they will taste).
10 Preheat the oven to 350ºF (175ºC).
11 Drain the chips and then mix in salt and pepper.
12 Arrange chips on greased baking sheet.
13 Bake for 30-35 minutes.
14 Enjoy!

Blueberry frozen yogurt recipes

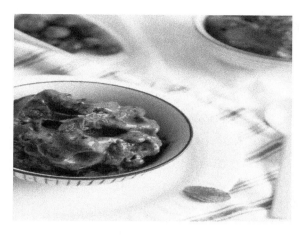

Ingredients

- 300 g blueberries frozen
- 150 g of yogurt at least 3.5% fat
- Sweetener and meringue to taste

Preparation

3 Puree frozen blueberries and yoghurt in a blender or with some stamina and a hand blender.
4 Fill in two bowls, lean back and enjoy.

Spicy avocado deviled eggs

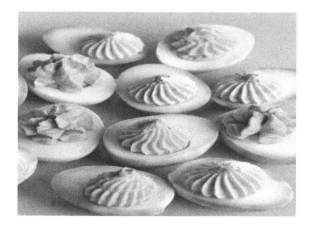

Ingredients *for about 8-10 egg halves*

Filling:

- 60 g organic salmon
- 60 g cream cheese
- 1 dash of lemon juice
- 60 g avocado
- 60 g cream cheese
- drops of lemon juice
- 100 g cream cheese
- 20 g pureed beetroot
- Salt / pepper
- Piment d'Espelette

For the colored eggs

- The broth from a
- large red cabbage, grated, boiled with a little water for 45 minutes.
- Juice of beetroot in the glass colored much stronger than my homemade puree
- 2 pieces of fresh turmeric, grated and boiled in 500 ml of water, the water is nice
- orange, remove the turmeric.

Preparation

16. Beat the hard-boiled eggs so that the shell is
17. cracked as evenly as possible. Place the eggs in each brew
18. and bathe in them for about 15-30 minutes.
19. No soda is first added to the red cabbage, some eggs are
20. dyed in it, and little bit of soda is gradually added until it reaches the
21. desired purple, blue and green shades.
22. Each salmon and avocado separately with the cream cheese with the
23. lightning hacker or blender puree and season with salt and pepper.
24. For the beetroot filling, add only so much puree that the
25. filling with the piping bag can be sprayed well, also season.
26. Fill all the fillings in the piping bag provided with the desired spouts
27. and either keep them cold or, when the eggs are completely
28. dyed, sprinkle them on.
29. Sprinkle all eggs with a pinch of Piment d'Espelette.
30. The eggs are still very handsome the next day, then discolored the avocado cream.

Sweet potato oat muffins

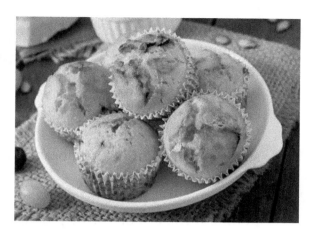

Ingredients

Dry ingredients:

- 150 g of ground oatmeal
- 75 g sugar of your choice
- 56 g of ground almonds
- 1/4 teaspoon soda
- pinch of salt
- 60 g milk-free chocolate chips and more for the top

Moist ingredients:

- 235 g of crushed sweet potato
- 160 ml of vegetable milk
- 1 tsp vanilla extract
- teaspoons vinegar

Preparation

9 Peel a medium sized sweet potato, cut into pieces / cubes and cook in water for about 10 minutes or until the pieces are soft (but not mushy). Drain the water and mash the sweet potato with a potato masher.

10 Preheat oven to 180 degrees C and lay a muffin dish with muffin paper or brush the inside of the molds with coconut oil. I used a silicone muffin mold.

11 Put all dry ingredients (except the chocolate chips) in a bowl and mix with a whisk. You can also process the dry ingredients in a sorler (I did that).

12 Add all wet ingredients and mix or mix in the Hexler until everything is mixed.

13 Finally, add the chocolate chips and stir with a spoon.

14 Spoon the dough into the muffin cups and spread more chocolate chips on top.

15 Bake in the oven for about 25 minutes or until a toothpick comes out clean. It's fine if the toothpick still comes out slightly sticky / crumbly, but it should not be wet.

16 Let the sweet potato muffins cool and enjoy!

Berry gummies Recipes

Currant butter cake from sheet metal

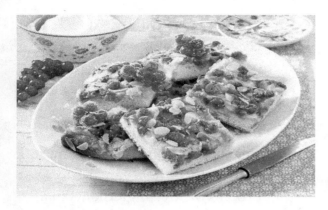

Ingredients *for 24 pieces*

- Fat and flour
- 200 ml of milk
- 1 cube (42 g) of fresh yeast
- 400 g of flour
- 75 g + 25 g + 2 tbsp sugar
- salt
- eggs (size M)
- 75 g + 225 g soft butter
- 500 g redcurrants
- 200 g of cold marzipan paste
- Flour
- 75 g almond flakes
- disposable syringe bag or small freezer bag

Preparation

7 Grease fat pan (about 32 x 39 cm, about 3.5 cm deep) and dust with flour. Warm the milk lukewarm. Break in the yeast and dissolve it. Mix flour, 75 g sugar, 1 pinch of salt, eggs and 75 g butter in little flakes in a bowl.

8 Add yeast milk and knead with the dough hook of the mixer. Cover in a warm place for about 45 minutes.

9 Read the berries, wash them and brush off the stems with a fork. Grate the marzipan roughly. Stir 225 g butter, marzipan and 25 g sugar creamy. Put in a disposable syringe bag.

10 Knead dough again. Dust with flour and roll out on the drip pan, pressing on the edge into the corners. Cover and let rise for about 20 minutes.

11 Press depressions into the dough with your thumbs or a thick wooden spoon. Cut off the tip of the piping bag. Spray marzipan paste into the wells. Distribute berries on the cake.

12 Sprinkle with almonds and 2 tablespoons of sugar. Bake in the preheated oven (electric cooker: 200 ° C / circulating air: 175 ° C / gas: see manufacturer) for 20-25 minutes. Allow to cool slightly.

Root mash recipes

Celery Root Mash

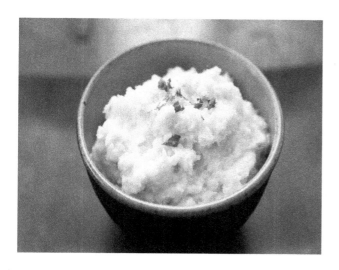

Ingredients

- pounds celery root
- 1/2 cup milk or cream
- tablespoons unsalted butter
- Salt to taste
- Chopped celery root leaves, for garnish (optional)

Preparation

6 Bring a large pot of salted water to a simmer (1 Tbsp of salt for every 2 quarts of water).

7 Peel and cube the celery root, boil until soft: While the water is coming to a boil, peel the celery roots with a knife. Cut the celery roots into 1-inch pieces.

8 Boil for 25-30 minutes, until soft.

9 Drain the pot, steam the celery root: Drain the pot, return the celery roots to the pot to the stovetop on low. Cover and let the celery roots steam for a minute or to, shaking the pan a bit to prevent sticking.

10 Add the milk or cream, butter and a generous pinch of salt and mash with a potato masher until it is as smooth as you like it. Add salt to taste and garnish with the celery root leaves, if using.

Lime-chili roasted cauliflower recipes

Chili and lime chicken with grilled sweet potato and cauliflower salad

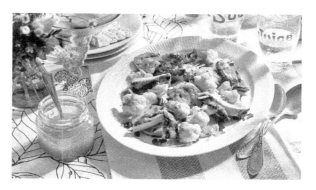

Ingredients *for 4 people*

- stalks / ciliary
- jalapenos
- cloves of garlic
- organic lime
- 1 tbsp and1 tsp liquid honey
- teaspoons and 1 pinch of salt
- 1 teaspoon chilli powder
- pieces (à 250 g) chicken fillet (with skin)
- 2 sweet potatoes
- small cauliflower
- 50 g almond sticks
- tbsp oil

- stalks / parsley
- 50 grams of almond paste
- 1 tablespoon of apple cider vinegar
- 1 teaspoon curry powder
- teaspoons of chilli sauce (eg Sriracha)
- pepper
- 50 g raisins

Preparation

6. Wash cilantro, shake dry. Peel leaves and chop finely. Wash, clean and finely chop jalapenos. Peel garlic and chop finely. Wash lime hot and rub dry. Rub the lime peel finely. Halve lime and squeeze juice. Juice, peel, coriander, jalapenos, garlic, 1 tablespoon honey, 2 teaspoons salt and 1 teaspoon chilli powder. Wash the meat, pat dry and mix with the marinade. Meat for about 2 hours.

7. Peel sweet potatoes, wash and cut into thin slices. Clean cauliflower, cut into small florets. Wash florets and drain well. Roast almonds in a frying pan without fat for about 3 minutes until golden brown and remove.

8. Heat 1 tbsp of oil in the pan. Cover with cauliflower and cook for 5-10 minutes. Then cook without lid for another 5-10 minutes until the cauliflower is golden brown.

9. Brush the grill with 1 tablespoon of oil, place the meat on the hot grill and cook until golden brown. Mix sweet potato slices and 2 tablespoons of oil. Place on the grill and grill on each side for 2-4 minutes until soft.

10. Wash parsley and shake dry. Peel leaves and chop finely. Almond flour, apple cider vinegar, 1 teaspoon honey, curry powder and chili sauce mix. Emplace 4 tbsp of oil. Season with salt and pepper. Remove meat and vegetables from the pan. Cut meat into strips. Serve meat, vegetables, almonds and raisins on plates. Sprinkle with parsley.

Cider-baked recipes

Frankfurt cider wreath

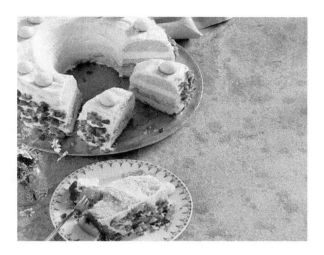

Ingredients *For 20 pieces*

- 200 g soft butter
- 1 tsp soft butter
- 1 pinch of salt
- 300 g of sugar
- tbsp sugar
- sachets of vanillin sugar
- eggs (size M)
- 225 g of flour
- 95 g cornstarch
- 1 packet of baking soda
- tablespoons milk
- sheets of gelatine
- apples
- Juice of 1 lemon
- 300 ml of cider
- 250 g of whipped cream
- 600 g double cream cream cheese
- 100 g dried soft apple rings
- Fat and breadcrumbs
- baking paper

Preparation

6   Mix 200 g of butter, salt, 200 g of sugar and 1 packet of vanillin sugar with the whisk of the hand mixer until creamy. Stir in eggs one after the other. Mix flour, 75 g of starch and baking powder and mix alternately with the milk under the fat-egg cream. Grease a ring mold (24 cm Ø, 2 liter content) well and sprinkle with breadcrumbs. Fill in the dough and smooth it out. Bake in preheated oven (electric cooker: 175 ° C / circulating air: 150 ° C / gas: see manufacturer) 35-40 minutes. Leave to cool on a wire rack for about 20 minutes. Drop out of the mold and allow to cool completely.

7   Soak the gelatine in cold water. Peel apples. Quarter 3 apples, cut out the core. Cut quarters into small pieces. In a pot with lemon juice and 150 ml of cider mix. Cover and simmer for about 5 minutes. Stir 50 ml of cider, 20 g of starch and 1 tbsp of sugar until smooth and stir in the compote, bring to a boil and allow to cool slightly.

8   Cut the cooled wreath 2x horizontally. Enclose lower bottom with a cake ring. Distribute the compote on top, place the middle of the tray and

leave to cool for approx. 15 minutes. Whip the cream. Cream cheese, 100 ml of cider, 100 g of sugar and 1 packet of vanilla sugar mix. Express gelatin, melt. Stir in 1-2 tablespoons cream cheese cream, then stir in the remaining cream. Fold in the cream. Leave the cream for about 15 minutes until it gets a little firmer.

9   Stir again with cream and coat about 1/3 of the cream on the middle ground. Put on the upper floor. Let it cool again for about 20 minutes. Remove the cake ring from the garland. Coat the wreath with the remaining cream all around. Cook the cake for about 2 hours. Dried apples cut into small cubes. Caramelise 4 tbsp sugar with 1 tbsp water in a small pan. Turn the apple cube into it and allow to caramelise for about 1 minute. Caramelised apples on a piece of baking paper, spread with the help of 2 forks and let cool.

10 Cut out balls from the rest of the apple using a ball cutter. Heat 1 tsp butter in a small pan, add apple balls, sprinkle with 1 tbsp sugar and deglaze with 1 tbsp water. Steam apple balls for about 2 minutes. Chop apple crisp small. Decorate cake with apple crisp and apple balls.

Tangy brussels sprout, onions and apple recipes

Brussels Sprouts With Apple

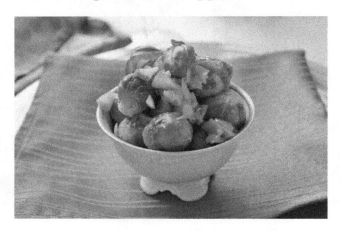

Ingredients *for 4 servings*

- stk Apple
- 500 G Brussels sprouts
- 1 prize salt
- EL Sunflower oil
- stk onions

Preparation

4   Wash and clean the Brussels sprouts. Mince the onions and let them turn glassy in oil.
5   Add water and add the Brussels sprouts. Make the whole thing simmer and add salt.
6   Peel and chop the apples and, after about 10 minutes cooking time, add the Brussels sprouts.

Easy roasted vegetables Recipes

Roasted vegetables with pomegranate

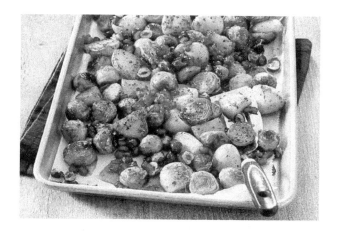

Ingredients *For 4 people*

- 800 g of small potatoes (triplets)
- 600 g Brussels sprouts
- tablespoons olive oil
- 1 teaspoon pepper flakes
- 1 teaspoon coarse sea salt
- pepper
- pomegranate (about 450 g)
- 75 g hazelnut kernels
- tablespoons of maple syrup

Preparation

3   Thoroughly wash the potatoes, grate them dry and halve, or quarter them. Brush, wash and halve Brussels sprouts. Mix potatoes and Brussels sprouts with oil, chili, salt and pepper in a bowl. Distribute the vegetables on a baking tray and roast in the preheated oven (electric cooker: 225 ° C / circulating air: 200 ° C / gas: see manufacturer) for approx. 25 minutes. Turn around once after about 15 minutes.

4   In the meantime halve the pomegranate and tap out the seeds with the help of a spoonful. Chop nuts roughly and add about 10 minutes before the end of the cooking time to the vegetables with maple syrup. Remove vegetables from the oven and sprinkle with pomegranate seeds.

Burst cherry tomatoes with garlic

Cherry Tomato Sauce

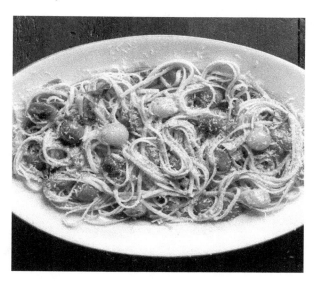

Ingredients

- 1 pound pasta
- Kosher salt
- 1/2 cup olive oil
- large garlic cloves, finely chopped
- pints cherry tomatoes
- 1/2 teaspoon freshly ground black pepper
- Pinch of sugar
- 1 cup coarsely chopped fresh basil

- Freshly grated Parmesan (for serving)

Preparation

4 Cook pasta in a large pot of boiling salted water, stirring occasionally, until al dente; drain and transfer to a large bowl.
5 Meanwhile, heat oil in a 12" skillet or wide heavy saucepan over medium-high. Add garlic, then tomatoes, pepper, sugar, and 1 tsp. salt. Cook, stirring occasionally, until tomatoes burst and release their juices to form a sauce, 6–8 minutes.
6 Toss pasta with tomato sauce and basil. Top with Parmesan.

Hummus-stuffed mini peppers Recipes

Simply barbecue: mini-peppers

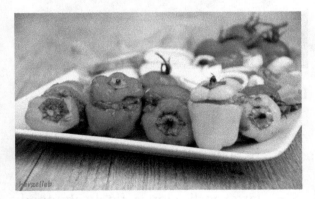

Ingredients

- 500 g ground beef
- 1 onion
- - 3 sprigs of thyme
- 1/2 cup of sour cream

- tablespoons of breadcrumbs
- 1-2 teaspoons salt
- pepper

Preparation

4 Finely chop the onion and the thyme and mix with the sour cream, salt and pepper under the minced meat. Add a little bit of breadcrumbs until the mass does not feel too moist.
5 Now you wash the peppers thoroughly, cut off the lid and remove the seeds. All you have to do is stuff the minced meat into the mini peppers and place them on the grill in a grill bowl.
6 Do not turn the peppers too fast and not too often, they may like to get a little brown, after all, the "roast aroma" is special in this dish.

Baked Zucchini fries recipes

Baked zucchini shells

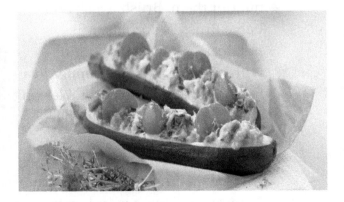

Ingredients

94

- small zucchini (à ca. 150 g)
- 2-3 spring onions
- fine sausages (approx. 100 g each)
- tablespoons butter
- Salt pepper
- some nutmeg
- 500 ml of vegetable stock
- Fat for the mold
- 125 g cherry tomatoes
- 70 g double-cream cheese
- 2-3 thyme branches

Preparation

6. Clean the zucchini and halve lengthwise. Carefully remove the inside with a spoon and chop. Clean the spring onions and cut into rings.
7. Sauté sausage from the sausages. Sauté with courgette heart and spring onions in hot butter, season with salt, pepper and nutmeg and allow to cool slightly.
8. Pre-heat the courgette halves in boiling broth for 3-5 minutes, drain. Place next to each other in a greased casserole dish. Wash cherry tomatoes and cut in half.
9. Pull cream cheese under the onion sausage mixture and season to taste, then add to the courgette halves. Press in the tomato halves. Remove thyme leaves from 1 branch, sprinkle over them.

10. Cook the courgette fish in a hot oven at 175 ° C for 30 minutes. Garnish with the remaining thyme.

Soups & Stews

bone broth

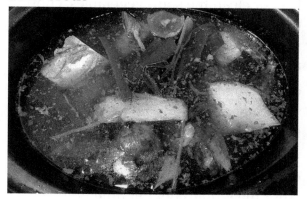

ingredients

2 kg Bovine bone (sand and marrow bones, mixed)
4 Onion (n)
6 liters Water, cold
4 tbsp Apple Cider Vinegar
2 cm ginger root
4 bay leaves
6 Allspice

preparation

Halve the onions and roast them together with the bones without adding fat in a large pot until everything has a nice dark color. Meanwhile, peel and quarter the ginger. Pour the bones in cold water, add the ginger, vinegar, bay leaves and allspice and bring to a boil. Adjust the stove so that the liquid stays at the boiling point. Allow to infuse for 18 - 24 hours. If you have the time, you can plan more, because only after 48 hours, all substances should be released from the bones.

Peel or clean the soup vegetables, chop them roughly and add them in the last two hours, then the vegetables should have given their complete taste. If it cooks longer, it could also taste bitter. The vinegar not only provides a round taste, but also serves to ensure that the ingredients are better able to dissolve out of the bones.

After the whole cooking time pour the soup through a sieve, dispose of bones and vegetables. Leave the broth a little and pour it over so gently that the (dirt collected on the bottom) "dirt" remains. Salt as desired.

This is the basic recipe. The broth can be drunk pure, expanded with meat and / or vegetables at will and serves as a strong base for many soups or sauces.

Ramen Base Broth:

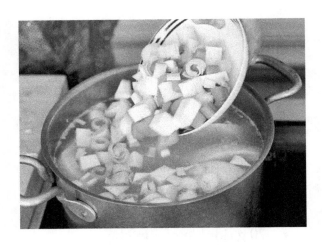

500 g Pork loin or pork loin
100 ml soy sauce
500 g Ramen noodles
4 toe / n garlic
3 Spring onions)
4 Carrot (n)
100 g bean sprouts
4 Egg (s)
1 pinch pepper
1 port. salt
1 tbsp sugar
4 Shiitake mushroom (s) or mushrooms
1 teaspoon Chilli flakes, at will
600 ml vegetable stock

preparation
The broth:
Put the soup chicken with a leek stick, an onion, three to four cloves of garlic, five centimeters of ginger in a piece, pinch of salt, three to four carrots and a handful of algae (optional) in cold water. Add so much water that the chicken is completely covered. (Choose a pot size that fits everything plus two to three

liters of water - a five liter pot is pretty good.)

Slowly bring to a simmer and simmer for at least 3 - 4 hours. Even more delicious is the broth at cooking times of 6 - 8 hours. Should foam arise you can skim this, but you do not have to.

The broth should not cook too much - only simmer lightly. The longer this broth cooks, the better. Then sift the broth. I do not continue using the cooked parts. It is worth to use a good and above all genuine soup chicken, not chicken.

The loin:

Sauté the pork loin in a pan briefly from all sides until it is slightly brownish. Do not fry for too long - only lightly brown! Then put in a pot and add 100 ml of soy sauce (I use Kikkoman because it is naturally brewed) and 50 to 100 ml of rice wine (I use Chinese rice wine). Add 1 tablespoon of sugar, a sliced spring onion (with the green and just a little of the onion) and 3 cm of grated fresh ginger. Add a little water so that the loin is almost completely covered with liquid. Then bring the liquid to a simmer. Again, just simmer gently.

After 40 minutes, remove the loin from the liquid and set aside. The loin before it comes into the soup, cut into approximately 2 - 3 mm thick slices. The loin should come from a good butcher - there are amazing quality differences. A good sirloin is very tender

and juicy after this procedure and not tough and dry.

The eggs:

cook and peel four eggs hard. Add the eggs to the loin stock and simmer for 10 minutes. Turn over and over so that they are evenly browned by the brew. When finished, halve and set aside.

The noodles:

You can make your own noodles while the broths are cooking or use Chinese vermicelli from Asiashop. I've had pretty good experiences with Quick-Noodles, but even spaghetti in it tastes very good. If you have a well-stocked shop, you may even get ramen noodles or fresh ramen noodles. The soup:

Cook the noodles but always strictly according to instructions and rather too hard than too soft. When the chicken broth is ready, place it together with the loin stock in a saucepan and season with a few tablespoons of soy sauce and another small shot of rice wine. Maybe even salting, but actually the soy sauce would have to provide enough salt. Then bring everything to a boil again. You can also add water, depending on how strong or diluted you want to have the soup. I leave the broth pure without adding water. When the soup is cooking, all other ingredients should be ready for the next step, especially the noodles. The garnish:

Brew the bean sprouts with hot water in a strainer. Cut the green of two spring onions into rings. Cut out of the Norib leaves small strips (about 2 x 3 cm).

The finish:

Put the soup in a bowl and add so many noodles that the noodles reach just below the surface.

Place two to three slices of loin. The loin can still be sprinkled with coarse pepper. Place half an egg with the yolk on the edge of the bowl.

Sprinkle a small handful of sprouts and spring onions over it and then put the nori leaf.

Enjoy the sight of the soup, preferably with chopsticks and sipping the broth - then it tastes best. Recipe:

GREEN MISO SOUP

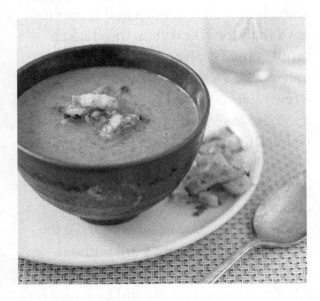

INGREDIENTS:

(gives: 4 servings)

2 tablespoons of grapeseed oil (or another neutral-tasting oil)

1 cup of finely chopped onions

4 cups vegetable stock or water

4 cups of chopped chard leaves (cut stems and leaf ribs first and set aside)

3 heaped tablespoons white or yellow miso paste

1 cup of chopped chard stalks and leaf ribs

2 tbsp breadcrumbs

PREPARATION:

1. Heat half of the oil at medium temperature in a saucepan. Fry the onions softly. Pour in the stock and heat until tender. Then add the chard leaves and cook for 3 minutes. Remove the pot from the heat, stir in the miso and finely puree the soup (if necessary in portions).

2. Heat the remaining oil in a small pan. Fry chard stalks and leaf ribs with the breadcrumbs in it for 1-2 minutes, stirring constantly, until the mixture becomes crispy.

3. Arrange the soup in preheated bowls and garnish with the crunchy mixture.

QUINOA MINESTRONE

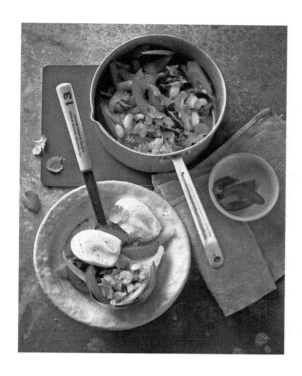

1 onion

1 clove of garlic

250 g of tomatoes

150 g of young zucchini

1 small carrot

100 g of celery

2 stems sage

2 tbsp olive oil

Sea or crystal salt

pepper

600 ml vegetable broth

60g quinoa

½ bunch of parsley

grated peel of ½ organic lemon

50 g freshly grated Parmesan

Peel and dice the onion and clove of garlic. The tomatoes scald, quench, skin and chop. Wash the zucchini, clean, halve lengthwise and slice. Peel the carrot, wash and clean the celery, cut both into slices. Wash, pluck and chop the sage leaves.

Heat the oil in a pot. Fry the onion and garlic in a glassy sauce. Add the vegetables, season with sage, salt and pepper. Add the broth, bring to the boil and sprinkle with the quinoa. Cover and cook for 15-20 minutes on a low heat.

Meanwhile, wash the parsley, shake it dry, pluck the leaves and chop. Mix with the lemon peel. Season the soup with salt and pepper, sprinkle with the parsley mixture and the Parmesan cheese on top.

Tip for the office: Fill the hot soup in a preheated thermo container, seal well - and enjoy lunch.

Spicy broccoli soup

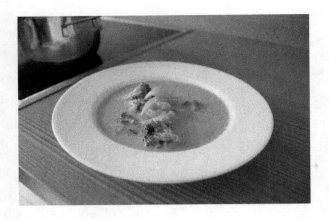

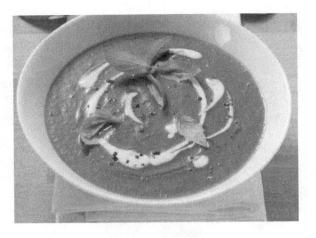

ingredients

1 Broccoli, fresh

1 Onion (n)

1 kl. Disk (s) Celery, fresh

1 pole / s leek

100 g cream cheese

½ TL Chilli flakes, dried

1 pinch Pepper, black, freshly ground

1 tbsp Parsley, dried

1 liter beef broth

preparation

Chop the onion, celery and leek and cook with the broccoli and spices in the beef broth for 20 minutes.

Add the melted cheese, let it melt for a short time and then puree it.

Creamy tomato soup

Ingredients

1 stk onion

1 Federation Suppengrün

1 EL oil

1 TL marjoram

1 TL Flour

0.5 l vegetable stock

1 can Tomatoes, peeled

1 prize salt

1 prize pepper

1 prize sugar

100 G whipped cream

preparation

For the creamy tomato soup, first remove the onion and finely dice. Then clean the soup vegetables and cut into small pieces.

Heat the oil in a saucepan and sauté the onion cubes and the soup vegetables with the marjoram for about 5 minutes.

Then add the flour and then with stirring the broth and stir the peeled tomatoes with juice - simmer for 15 minutes.

Then finely puree the soup with the blender, stir in the whipped cream and season with salt, pepper and sugar.

Cauliflower soup

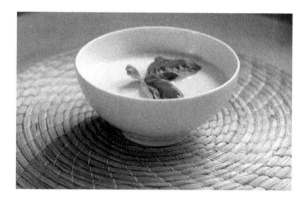

Ingredients: for 4 people

1 medium cauliflower (600 g)

750 ml water

1 level tsp salt

150 ml milk (1,5% fat)

100 ml sweet cream (30% fat)

1 tablespoon flour stock cubes (finished product)

salt

white pepper

Toasted bread cubes:

4 slices Toasted bread

1 heaped tsp butter (15 g)

parsley to sprinkle

Picture of cauliflower soup

Click on picture to enlarge

Preparation:

For the cauliflower soup recipe, first clean the cauliflower, cut into florets, wash and strain in a sieve.

Put salted water and milk in a saucepan and bring to a boil.

You should not lose sight of the pot, as the milk overcooks too much heat.

Put the cauliflower florets into the boiling liquid, bring to the boil again, then slowly boil the cauliflower in about 20 minutes.

Remove the pot, blend the cauliflower with the liquid using a hand blender, or squeeze the whole mixture through a strainer.

Mix the flour with the cream in a small bowl, stir into the cauliflower soup, and at the same time add a broth cube to the pan.

Put the pan back onto the hot plate and boil the cauliflower soup thoroughly with a whisk, stirring gently, then cook for about 5 minutes. Now is the moment where you can extend the amount of cauliflower soup, as desired.

If desired, add some more broth or water and thicken with a little extra flour.

Finally, season the cauliflower soup to taste with some salt and white ground pepper.

Sprinkle the cauliflower soup with plenty of fresh parsley, serve.

Roasted bread cubes taste very good with this simple, home-style cauliflower soup.

For the preparation of roasted bread cubes, Cut the toast into small cubes, place in a coated frying pan, without additional fat, and roast the bread cubes round tenderly golden-yellow to light-brown with constant use of a spatula.

Pull the pan aside and only then add 1 heaped tsp butter to the pan and turn the still hot croutons into it.

In this way you get crispy, tasting wonderful butter, relatively low-fat roasted bread cubes.

Serve the bread cubes with the cauliflower soup.

Shchi

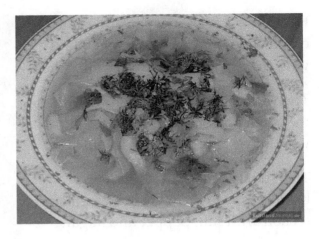

Ingredients

2 l water

200 g Soupmeat

750 g (or a small head) white cabbage

3 onions

1 big each Carrot and tomato (or 1 tbsp tomato paste)

2 potatoes

1 teaspoon Caraway seed

2 bay leaves

10 black peppercorns

4 Garlic cloves

2 tablespoons each Parsley and dill

200 g sour cream

Salt pepper

Put the meat on little water (enough to cover the meat), heat it up and bring it to a boil until it forms foam. Pour away the water and remove the foam residue from the pot. Refill the meat with hot water, bring to the boil, add a whole onion, 2 cloves of garlic and bay leaves and cook over low heat for about 2 hours.

Throw away the cooked onion and bay leaves from the broth. Remove meat and cut it to size.

Shchi preparation

Remove white cabbage from outer leaves, cut out the stump. Grate cabbage.

Finely dice the remaining 2 onions and garlic. Cut the potato into fine strips. Grate carrot.

Put everything together with the white cabbage in the boiling meat broth (or boiling water) and cook on low heat for 15 minutes.

Wash tomato, cut into quarters and add to the soup with peppercorns and cumin. Simmer for another 10 minutes.

When the meat has been removed from the broth, it will also come into the pot about 5 minutes before the end of cooking.

Season the cabbage soup with salt and pepper.

Sprinkle shchi with plenty of parsley and dill and serve with plenty of sour cream (about 2 tablespoons each).

Fast Red Lentil Dal

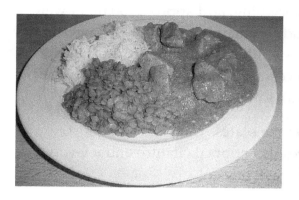

ingredients

1 Onion (s), diced

1 Garlic clove (s), chopped

1 tbsp Ginger, chopped

something oil

3 cups / n Lentils, red

something yogurt

something coriander leaves

something Onion (s), (onion rings)

½ TL salt

1 teaspoon, heaped turmeric

1 ½ tsp curry powder

½ TL Spice mixture, (Garam Masala)

preparation

Heat some oil in a saucepan, sauté onions, garlic and ginger. Then add all the spices except salt and roast, stir well so it does not matter. Now come the lenses. I take coffee cups, not pots. Mix everything, add approx. 250 ml of water and simmer for approx. 15 minutes until the lentils are soft, but not mushy, if necessary. Add some more water. Season with salt until finally.

On the plates, Then make yoghurt, freshly chopped cilantro and a few onion rings in one go.

BUTTERNUT CREAM SOUP WITH COCONUT MILK

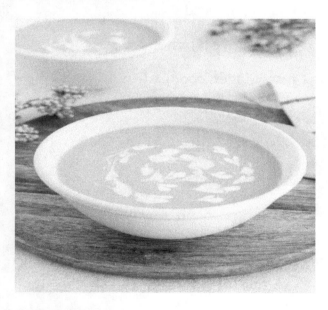

INGREDIENTS

• 1200 g of butternut squash

• 2 garlic cloves

• 2 onions

• 1 tablespoon butter

• salt + freshly ground pepper

• about 1/2 teaspoon cayenne pepper

• some chili from the mill* or a few chilli flakes

• 2 tsp turmeric

• 700 ml vegetable broth

• 800 ml coconut milk

• 1 tbsp lemon juice

• fresh coriander or fresh parsley to taste

PREPARATION:

Peel the butternut squash and cut into small pieces. Peel garlic cloves and onion and chop finely. Melt the butter in a large saucepan and sauté the butternut for 2 to 3 minutes. Add onion and garlic and fry for another 4 to 5 minutes. Season with salt, pepper, cayenne, chili and turmeric. Add vegetable broth and coconut milk and simmer for about 20 minutes until the butternut is tender. Puree the butternut cream soup with the blender and season with lemon juice, salt and pepper. Wash coriander or parsley, shake dry and chop, if necessary. Serve with the butternut cream soup.

Vegetable soup with herbal turkey balls

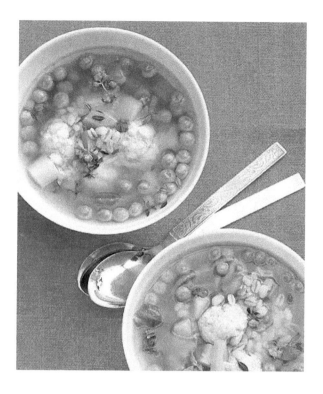

Ingredients:

- 400 g turkey breast;
- 2 potatoes;
- 1 onion;
- 1 carrot;
- 200 g of cauliflower;
- 170 g of frozen green peas;
- ½ small bunch of parsley;
- 1, 5 liters. water
- 2 TBSP. l small pasta;
- 2 TBSP. l sunflower oil;

- 1 tsp salts;
- ¼ tsp. black pepper

Cook

1. Wash the cauliflower and divide it into small twigs. Chop the onion, dice the potatoes and grate the carrot. Wash parsley and chop.

2. Pour oil into a deep pan and heat it. Add the onion to the hot oil and lower slightly, then add the carrot, mix and fry until the ingredients are tender.

3. Put the potato cubes in a saucepan, add water, place on the heat, bring to a boil and cook.

4. Wash turkey breast, chop, season with salt and pepper, sprinkle with parsley and mix well. From the cooked filling with wet hands form small meatballs.

5. Add all the meatballs to the boiling soup one at a time and stir gently with a spoon so that nothing sticks together. Season the salted soup and cook for 3-4 minutes.

6. After this time, add cauliflower twigs and frozen peas to the soup and cook for 5 minutes. Then lay out the onion with the carrot and boil for another 5 minutes.

7. At the end of cooking, add the pasta and, if necessary, add salt (universal seasoning). Boil the soup for a few

minutes, remove from the heat, cover and leave to rest for about 20 minutes.

8. After 20 minutes put the soup with turkey meatballs in a plate and serve with bread, vegetables and vegetables.

Avocado Chicken Soup

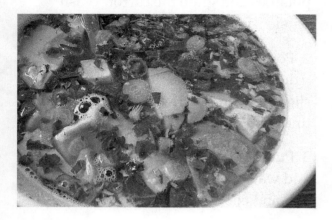

ingredients

300 g Chicken breast

1 Avocado (s)

2 Spring onions)

1 handful coriander leaves

700 ml broth

1 toe garlic

1 Lime (n)

something oil

salt and pepper

preparation

Heat the oil (if you like it a bit more hot, take chilli oil) in a saucepan, lightly salt the chicken breast and fry gently all around. Once it's through, take out of the pot.

Now cut the spring onions into fine rings and add to the hot oil, sauté briefly, then squeeze the garlic.

Shortly before the garlic begins to brown, deglaze with the broth.

Now tear the chicken breast into the smallest possible pieces and put it back into the soup. Squeeze out the lime and add the juice to the soup.

Remove the avocado from the skin and cut into pieces that are not too small, divide them on two large soup bowls, season with salt and pepper, add the hot soup and sprinkle with coarsely chopped coriander leaves.

Anti-Inflammatory Diet

for Beginners

The Complete Guide to Heal the Immune System, Manage the Symptoms

of Inflammation, Restore Optimal Health with Easy Foods and Meal Plan

Solutions to Feel Better

By Claire K. McLoss

Table of Contents

Introduction **110**

Chapter 1: What Is Inflammatory Disease **111**

Inflammation and Overall Health: *113*

Distinguishing Inflammatory Disease from Other Illnesses *116*

Diagnoses of Inflammatory Disease and your Next Steps: *116*

Chapter 2: Resolving Anti-Inflammatory Disease **121**

Anti-Inflammatory Diet *121*

Benefits of the Diet *124*

Different types of food that are part of the Anti-Inflammatory Diet *125*

Foods to avoid *128*

Chapter 3: History of the Anti-Inflammatory Diet **131**

Chapter 4: The Diet and You **134**

Chapter 5: Tasty meals **138**

Chapter 6: Traveling with the Anti-Inflammatory Diet **145**

Mediterranean: *145*

India: *148*

Mexican/Hispanic Food/Latin: *150*

Asian Food: *152*

Italian: *153*

Chapter 7: Setting Up A Schedule: Taking Action **157**

Sunday: *157*

Monday: *158*

Tuesday: *160*

Wednesday: *161*

Thursday:.. *163*

Friday:... *165*

Saturday:.. *167*

Chapter 8: The Popular Diet **169**

Mike Tyson: *170*

Kevin Smith: *171*

Penn Jillette: *171*

Hannah Teter: *172*

David Haye: *172*

Barney Du Plessis: *172*

Nate Diaz: *173*

Meagan Duhamel *173*

Gama Pehalvan: *173*

Venus Williams: *173*

Scott Jurek: *174*

Jermain Defoe: *174*

Ellen DeGeneres: *174*

Usher: *174*

Conclusion **176**

Description **177**

Introduction

Congratulations on purchasing *Anti-Inflammatory Diet for Beginners* and thank you for doing so. A common ailment which has become a serious problem for people's health and well-being is an inflammatory disease. Dangerous on its own and dangerous when left unchecked. Inflammation is a common process and protective mechanism for our bodies, however, when inflammation gets out of hand, it can lead to an inflammatory disease which can have detrimental health consequences for all us. It is a disease that can ravage the body and create permanent issues and even be fatal. For this reason, it is important to understand the disease and how to deal with it by eating a proper anti-inflammatory diet. It is crucial to our daily well-being.

While there are many medical and lifestyle changes a person may make in order to improve or even resolve inflammation, in this book, we will mainly be discussing diet and its effects on this particular disease process. We will be discussing what causes inflammation, the signs and symptoms to look out for, and what dietary steps one can take in order to minimize, prevent, and even resolve the effects of inflammatory disease. The information provided will give a solid understanding of how the food we ingest has a positive or negative impact on the inflammatory disease process and our health. Simple, everyday changes to our routine can improve our overall health and well-being in ways we can't even imagine. Diet can be used as a very strong tool in order to put those affected by this often-debilitating disease on the right path.

The inflammatory diet is a diverse diet which can improve the health and livelihoods of many people suffering from a painful and often deadly disease. With this particular diet, we may have to skimp on some ingredients, but hopefully not on taste and definitely not on nutrients. A healthy diet which still satisfies our palate is what we will be discussing.

Through this book, we hope to be able to answer any questions or concerns about what inflammatory disease is, as well as what steps people can take in order to prevent or improve the signs and symptoms through a well-balanced diet. With the information provided, people suffering from the inflammatory disease can still live relatively normal and active lives as long as they are willing to make the effort. The first step is in knowing; the second is in making the changes that are necessary. After all, knowledge without action is ultimately meaningless. Knowledge is power. Action is essential. Let's learn about some great eating habits, and then go out there and enjoy what the world has to offer.

There are plenty of books on this subject on the market, thanks again for choosing this one! Every effort was made to ensure it is full of as much useful information as possible, so please enjoy!

Chapter 1: What Is Inflammatory Disease

Before we can fully appreciate the anti-inflammatory diet and what it does, we must understand what it is used to prevent and the process of chronic inflammation. Chronic inflammation is basically a normal body process that goes unchecked. Inflammation, on its surface, is not a bad thing. In fact, it is essential for our bodies in order to maintain health and prevent being overcome by ravaging disease. It is not an illness in and of itself, but a natural response by our immune system to illness, infection, and foreign substances that enter the body. When our own immune system feels threatened by something it does not recognize, it jumps into action with an inflammatory response, which results in an increase in white blood cells, immune cells, and cytokines to the affected area. When the immune system feels threatened, it jumps into action. This response is a normal way for the body to protect itself. Basically, like our own army fighting off an outside invader. The fact is that inflammatory responses are occurring inside of us constantly and we don't even realize it. It is amazing how our bodies have multiple metabolic processes going on inside of us to keep us healthy and to keep us running. All without us even knowing. The human body is truly a specimen of great functions in and of itself. For this reason alone, we should treat our bodies with the very best care that we can. Our bodies truly are a temple, to recite an old adage.

Think about when you get a cut. The affected area can become red, swollen, and warm. Our body temperature may also rise. These are the result of various immune cells and body processes helping us fend off an attack from a foreign substance that does not naturally occur in our bodies. When injuries to our body occur, such as with a cut, the damaged cells release multiple chemicals that cause blood vessels to leak fluid into the tissues, which in turn, causes swelling. The chemicals released during this whole process also attract white blood cells and other immune cells to the area which basically eat up and eliminate the injury-causing substance and also eat the dead cells. The white blood cells that eat up everything are called phagocytes. Phagocytes eventually die after completing their job. In most circumstances, the inflammation is short-lived and goes down after the threat has been subdued. If you experience mild inflammation, know that your body and immune system are doing their job to keep you protected from harmful diseases. An external wound and the swelling we witness is a much more visual representation of inflammation that we can actually observe. Similar operations are going on inside of us that we can't physically see. It is a complicated and in-depth process, indeed. But our immune systems are designed to take care of it.

Think about it this way: An unwanted and dangerous person walks into your house, with the intent of doing severe damage. Imagine also that there is some type of security system in the home. Everyone inside is alerted of the breach and they immediately jump into action. The vicious guard dogs pounce on the person, the people come in and subdue the culprit, and then throw them out of the house. The police come and take them away. A couple of household items get damaged in the process, but as a whole, the dangerous threat has been taken care of. The people and the dogs stop fighting when they no longer need to, and things begin getting back to normal. The small damage that was done to the house will slowly get repaired by the people inside. No harm, no foul.

What the heck is the point of this story? It illustrates our own immune system protecting us from harmful invaders. The dogs and the people in the home represent the immune cells pouncing on and fighting off the unwanted substance, represented by the unwelcome intruder. Just like with the story, once a threat to our bodies is eliminated, under normal circumstances, our internal body processes go back to normal. The inflammatory process is complete. We hope that in the situation with the home, nobody dies. Believe it or not, the inflammation that occurs in our bodies is much more violent. Cells are actually dying. Someone should make an animated action movie about this whole process. Perhaps it can be called "Inflammation Army". Well, that's not too creative, but it could become the next big thing.

In more extreme situations, the inflammation may be misdirected, and this can lead to inflammatory disease, which is a serious illness. This is when the inflammatory response can become a problem. In these cases, the immune system will begin attacking healthy tissues and organs, rather than diseased ones. Our internal immune cells will jump into action, but there is nothing to fight. If there is no pathogen, then what gets attacked? Our own body, and if it's not dealt with early, it can cause severe damage. Rheumatoid arthritis is an example of a result of chronic inflammatory disease. This disease can be characterized by painful, warm, stiff, and swollen joints. In most cases of mild inflammation, this is temporary. With rheumatoid arthritis, it is long term and can become permanent. Other examples of chronic inflammatory disease include asthma, tuberculosis, Crohn's disease, lupus, and periodontitis, which is major gum disease. Remember when your dentist told you that oral disease may be indicative of overall health? Well, they weren't lying. No matter how much we want to avoid it, it is important to go to the dentist for regular checkups.

While the inflammatory disease is most often associated with the joints, in more extreme cases, other organs, including vital internal organs, of the body can be affected. Signs and symptoms are based on which part of the body is under attack. Long term and untreated inflammation can lead to detrimental health consequences. It is important to understand that chronic inflammation that can be assessed on the outside can also be indicative of internal inflammatory disease. This is the point we really want to drive home, and we will be doing it constantly, because it is our health, after all. We don't just want to increase our longevity in life, but our quality of life also.

Let's go back to the story from earlier. In that scenario, there was an unwanted intruder, and everyone inside the home jumped into action to subdue and eliminate the threat. This is inflammation at its finest. A threat was perceived, the proper alarms were initiated, and everyone involved jumped into action and did what they were supposed to do. Our immune system army is probably the most organized team we can imagine. Not only that, it works around the clock and never takes a break. If it ever does, that's when we are in trouble. Now, imagine that the same thing occurs as far as the people and the dogs in the home. The difference now is, there is no intruder. For whatever reason, everybody inside the home rushes to the front door area and begins fighting and attacking the area. There is nothing to attack though. They just keep going and start damaging the home and all of the items inside of it. Also, since there was no threat in the first place, there is nothing to indicate to anyone to stop fighting. So, everyone just keeps going and continues to damage the home, until there is literally nothing left. There was no reason for them to do what they did and no one to stop them either. The home is destroyed, maybe even beyond repair. This is what can happen to our bodies with chronic and uncontrolled inflammatory disease. With enough time, our bodies can be completely damaged. Let's make sure this does not happen to us. Let's figure out ways to stop this. We are here for you and your health. We hope you enjoyed this story. There are plenty more to come.

Inflammation and Overall Health:

Chronic Inflammation, no matter where it is, can affect our overall health and well-being. First of all, let's discuss the physical impacts of the pain and swelling, as with rheumatoid arthritis. This can severely limit our physical capabilities, impact our work and our hobbies, and just create a miserable day-to-day experience. When we wake up in pain, it puts a damper on the rest of our day. When we experience pain throughout the day, it limits our movement, our work ethic, our relationships, and our overall ability to enjoy life. It is difficult to deal with this kind of pain for a day, let alone day after day with no improvement in sight. Imagine being a grandparent and you just want to wake up in the morning and take your grandkids to the park. You would love to just be able to wake up, get ready, and go have some fun. When you wake up though, your knees, your hips, and your back are aching to the point that you can barely move, let alone go anywhere. This creates a huge impact on our lifestyle. Many peoples' mobility becomes so poor that they cannot get around without the aid of a device, like wheelchair or walker. Other people can barely get out of bed and become sedentary. Pain and swelling, indeed, wreak havoc on our everyday lives no matter how tough we think we are. Some pain and immobility are a result of natural aging. However, a lot of it can be avoided by making simple lifestyle changes. Some things in life are beyond our control. It is best that we do not waste time worrying about them and deal with things as they come. Worrying about a problem is often worse than dealing with the problem itself. However, as far as the things we can control, we should try our best to do so.

With illnesses like rheumatoid arthritis, pain can hit from anywhere at any time with little to no warning. You could be asleep in the middle of the night, cooking in the kitchen, or working at your job. Suddenly, out of nowhere, debilitating pain hits you and takes you out of commission. This pain can become so bad for people that they have to be rushed to the hospital. Sometimes, the pain is localized to a certain area, other times, it is widespread throughout the body. It is a debilitating pain beyond what we can imagine unless we have personally dealt with it. It may sound like hyperbole, but it is anything but that. Pain and immobility from chronic inflammation is nothing to take lightly.

Furthermore, inflammatory disease can impact our health depending on which part of the body is being impacted. All of the organs and organ systems are at risk. Here are some examples.

- Inflammation of the heart, which is called myocarditis, can lead to fluid retention and difficulty breathing. This will ultimately lead to a lack of perfusion of oxygen-rich blood and excess fluid in the body will eventually have a detrimental effect on other vital organs. Widespread swelling throughout the body, often called edema, creates pressure and excessive workload on the heart and many other vital organs. If prolonged, extreme wear and tear will occur. Our heart can only function under these conditions for so long before the muscle starts shutting down. Heart disease, congestive heart failure, heart attack, poor contractility, sudden cardiac arrest, and risk of stroke all increase in probability with unchecked inflammatory disease. Who would have ever thought that chronic joint pain could also be indicative of heart disease? The truth of the matter is, it can. So, take it seriously.

- Inflammation of the airways can lead to difficulty breathing and damage to the lungs. This will, in turn, decrease the oxygen-rich blood available to perfuse the rest of the body. Pneumonia, pulmonary (lung) edema, chronic obstructive pulmonary disease, respiratory failure, and a wealth of other respiratory system illnesses will result from an inflammatory disease that is not taken care of early. When your breathing is affected, your life is affected. Oxygen is a life force, and we need it all of the time.

- Inflammation of the kidneys, nephritis, can lead to kidney failure and impact many functions of the body including blood pressure regulation and fluid and electrolyte balance. Our kidneys are often not given the credit they deserve, like the brain, heart, or lungs. However, the kidneys perform a lot of functions beyond what was just mentioned earlier. When our kidneys fail, our bodies cannot properly eliminate excess fluid and toxins that come from what we eat and drink and through normal metabolic functions. Almost everything we ingest gets processed by our kidneys. There is also a lot of breakdowns that occur in our bodies through various metabolic processes. If these broken-down substances remain in our bodies for too long, they can become toxic. All of these waste products are eliminated by our kidneys. To bring it full circle, when our kidneys cannot eliminate waste, which is essentially what urine is, then the buildup in our bodies will impede on our heart, lungs, brain, and other organs. Our bodies will not utilize calcium properly, leading to bone disease. And our red blood cell production will go down, too. If we go into kidney failure, immediate medical response is needed, up to and including, dialysis or a kidney transplant. Poor kidneys equal poor health. The most frightening part is, symptoms from kidney disease may not manifest until it is way too late. That is why the earliest signs and symptoms must be taken seriously. Fatigue, muscle stiffness, pain, and swelling are all early warning signs that there could be a problem. See how important our kidneys are?

- Inflammation of the digestive tract can lead to severe issues such as diarrhea, bloody stools, fatigue, and unintended weight loss. Yes, unintended weight loss is not a good thing no matter how you want to spin it. The digestive disease should not be a diet plan. Digestive tract health is often overlooked, but it is essential to our well-being. This might get a little gross for some but think about when you have been constipated for days. You feel fatigued, bloated, irritable, and just plain miserable. Then one day, you have a huge bowel movement. Suddenly, you feel so much better. It is a pretty amazing feeling to have after the fact. This is a simple example, but yes, digestive tract health is very important. The digestive system breaks down the food that we eat and absorbs and assimilates it into our bodies. Food that is not absorbed eventually gets eliminated. This process of digestion is very in-depth and very important to the functionality of our bodies. Also remember, the digestive system is not just our stomach and intestines. It also includes many ancillary organs like the liver, gallbladder, and pancreas. A poor functioning digestive system will affect a multitude of other body processes. For chronic digestive issues, seek the help of professionals to see if there is anything concerning going on. It may be a simple solution, or it could be something more complicated. Make sure to find out. Take the time you need for your health.

Remember that all of our organs and systems work in conjunction with one another. They have their own unique functions, but the functions of one intensely affect the others. Some have a much more mutualistic relationship, like the heart and lungs. Others have a more secondary or tertiary relationship. In the end, if one is affected, they can all become affected. This is especially true if inflammation persists for an extended period of time. It is important to recognize the early signs and symptoms of inflammation and seek help immediately. Let's not wait until we need a heart transplant or dialysis to begin taking our health seriously. This may sound extreme, but in the end, it is still a reality. Remember the house that got destroyed? Don't let yourself be that house. We don't want to provide this information to scare you. We don't want you to get up each day and be terrified of what can happen. On the contrary, we want you to have more peace of mind knowing that your health is being taken care of. Don't worry about the things you can't control and work hard on the things you can. Your personal health is something you have control over.

Distinguishing Inflammatory Disease from Other Illnesses

While the inflammatory disease may have distinct signs and/or symptoms. It can also mimic other illnesses as well. With inflammation, people may experience flu-like symptoms like a headache, chills, and muscle stiffness. Many of the signs/symptoms we spoke about earlier may or may not be caused by inflammatory disease. With continued research though, it has been determined that many of our illnesses are caused by chronic inflammation. Whatever the case, seek medical attention for any of these health concerns. Chronic or extended inflammation is not something you want to take lightly.

Diagnoses of Inflammatory Disease and your Next Steps:

Various diseases that occur can produce similar signs and symptoms for a person. We never truly know what illness we have until we have certain diagnostic exams performed on us. Before we go there though, let's get more in-depth about the various manifestations of inflammatory disease. If you are experiencing these on a regular basis, then it's time to make some serious changes.

- One of the most common symptoms of inflammatory disease is swelling. With the influx of white blood cells, the fluid from these cells needs to go somewhere, so it begins pooling in certain areas of the body. More often than not, this will be in the joints and extremities. Due to gravity, a lot of the time, the swelling will occur in the feet or lower extremities. Walking long distances can have a major impact on this. In addition, fluid collection swelling may occur in the neck, back, and shoulder area and cause chronic pain here as well. This can also be related to lifestyle or stress and injury, but it is important to get confirmation if it is chronic pain. If chronic pain can be avoided, then why live with it? In many cases, you may not have to deal with it at all.

- Headache, fatigue, chills, weakness, and muscle soreness or stiffness are common symptoms of inflammatory disease. They may mimic a cold or flu, but it is important to get it diagnosed for sure, especially if they are chronic issues. If a person has these symptoms regularly, but otherwise healthy, it is a strong indication of inflammatory disease. These are also some of the earlier warning signs, so a good time to get checked out.

- There has been much research in the past that inflammation can directly affect our mood, resulting in mood swings and depression. For example, people with heart disease who also appeared to be depressed generally had higher inflammation levels with lab testing. Feeling down and don't know why, maybe it's not your fault, but something you can control physically. And let's be real, when we feel healthy, we often feel happier. Continued research is coming out that shows the correlation between physical health and mental health. Many clinicians and mental health professionals are working together to determine some of the correlations between the two. For example, the disciplines of neurology and psychiatry are merging together in many ways to understand the strong relationship between mood and physical health. There is strong support to even merge these two disciplines together completely. Whatever the case, just realize that a poor daily mental outlook may be indicative of poor physical health. If you are always in a poor mood, seek the help of a professional. Maybe there is something that can be done about it.

- Inflammatory disease can commonly cause issues with the skin. Skin inflammation will manifest with itchiness, redness, rashes, and even chronic conditions like dermatitis. It may be as simple as needing a better moisturizer, or it could be something much more concerning. Skin issues are another thing that is taken lightly. There have been many sitcoms in the past that have even insulted the specialty of dermatology. The jokes are actually pretty funny. However, nothing could be farther from the truth. Our skin is our largest organ. It covers our whole body and has so many different layers. It serves more functions than we can imagine. It is also usually the first line of defense from outside invaders. Skin health can also be a strong determinant in assessing general health. Chronic illnesses may manifest themselves on the skin first. For example, Lupus, which is another inflammatory/auto-immune disease, may manifest itself on the skin with certain types of circular rashes. Furthermore, dry and itchy skin can be indicative of kidney disease. These may be an extreme example, but one of the goals of this eBook is to help the reader understand how inflammatory disease can present itself. Do not take skin conditions lightly. They are a strong indicator of our overall health and wellness. Some good news regarding the skin as it relates to the anti-inflammatory diet, which we will discuss later on. Many dermatologists maintain that an anti-inflammatory will give you smoother and younger-looking skin. This may sound like a commercial for moisturizer, but it is true that various types of food have an effect one way or another on the skin.

- Inflammation can create very painful and uncomfortable symptoms in the digestive tract. Acid reflux, bloating, and diarrhea can occur due to inflammation. Abdominal pain and cramping can also become very severe. Crohn's disease is an anti-inflammatory bowel disease that affects the lining of the digestive tract. If left unchecked, it can cause life-threatening complications. We talked earlier about not taking digestive tract health lightly. Not only can so many diseases affect the digestive tract, poor digestive health heavily weighs down on our lifestyles. Imagine sitting at a ball game and having to get up every few minutes to use the restroom. Imagine being at a restaurant or other gathering and not being able to sit still due to digestive problems. This is certainly no way to live. A proper diet can really have a positive result for our digestive tract. We will discuss this later. For now, let's continue further with inflammatory disease.

- Heart and lung disease are associated with inflammation. Studies from top universities have found that coronary artery disease risks have a strong connection to inflammation. Many different cardiac diseases will result from inflammation. Also, asthma, chronic obstructive pulmonary disease, infections, and many other pulmonary diseases are associated with lung inflammation. This can also lead to fluid accumulation, which will result in breathing difficulties. We discussed earlier the correlation between inflammatory disease and the heart and lungs. We really want to emphasize the severity of its impact. The heart and lungs also have a strong mutual relationship with each other as they are constantly feeding each other blood and other substances directly. The heart sends blood to the lungs to receive its oxygen supply, and then the lungs send the oxygen-rich blood back to the heart to pump to the rest of the body. Their relationship is truly symbiotic. Do you have chest pain, difficulty breathing, fatigue, swelling in the feet, or other symptoms of concern? Get checked out immediately.

- Chronic inflammatory disease can also lead to a decrease in bone density. Higher risks of osteoporosis and fractures will result from a lack of bone growth. It may be hard to recognize the signs and symptoms here, but oftentimes, it can be excessive back pain, loss of height, or fracturing a bone with even mild trauma. We hope that if you fracture something, you will go to the hospital anyway. Upon arriving at the hospital, a healthcare provider should ask you how you received a fracture.

If it was from a trauma that was not that severe, then further tests for inflammation can be done. We touched on the effects of inflammatory disease as it relates to the musculoskeletal system with the swelling of the joints and extremities. Let's delve more into how it can affect the system overall. Inflammatory disease can cause any of a group of diseases called myopathies. In short, myopathy is an umbrella term used to describe a multitude of conditions affecting the muscles. There are several different types of myopathies, but the primary symptom with all of them is muscle weakness. Myopathies may produce simple effects like weakness, fatigue, or mild pain. However, in a more extreme case, severe debilitation may occur and things can also become fatal such as when it affects the muscles that help us swallow or help us breathe. Take even the mildest forms of musculoskeletal disease seriously, especially if they are chronic.

While many of these signs and symptoms are indicative of inflammatory disease, we cannot be certain until certain diagnostic exams are completed. While many advanced clinicians would most likely be able to tell by the signs and symptoms you are having, they cannot be sure until further testing is done. As we said, many types of diseases can produce similar symptoms. Word of advice: do not go to your healthcare worker friend and ask them to diagnose you by what you tell them. They will not be able to tell you for sure. First of all, a thorough examination by a healthcare provider is essential. They will do a physical assessment to check on the swelling, plus ask in-depth questions about lifestyle, symptoms of pain, what you have been experiencing, and how long your current issues have been going on. The physical assessment will really be focused on your joints and extremities. Likely, they will check your mobility, doing a neurological assessment, and check your vital signs. By doing a thorough examination, the healthcare provider can help to distinguish between inflammatory disease and other ailments. One of the biggest indicators of chronic illness as related to joint pain and swelling is by knowing how long it has been going on and if the signs and symptoms are getting worse.

Furthermore, diagnostic tests such as scans, which include x rays, ultrasounds, CT scans, or MRIs may be needed to assess internal issues related to inflammation. An MRI, especially with some type of contrast agent, is the most in-depth of the scans. Also, certain blood tests will likely be performed to check for certain markers related to inflammatory disease. A common blood test used to assess inflammatory disease is C-Reactive Protein, a major marker indicative of inflammation found on blood tests. We will talk more about C-reactive proteins later on. All of these assessment strategies will work in congruency with one another to get the most comprehensive information needed to make a proper diagnosis. Without these, there is truly no way of knowing for sure what ails us.

As you can see, inflammatory disease can have detrimental effects on the body, including many vital organs. For this reason, it is important to recognize the signs and symptoms and seek treatment immediately. Many people may call you a hypochondriac, but it is ultimately your health and not there's. Care must be taken in order to get the correct diagnosis and start a proper treatment plan, the backbone of which is a proper diet.

We hope that this chapter has given you a solid understanding of the inflammatory disease. While the inflammatory disease can be damaging to our health, with proper care and recognition, the negative results can be minor or even nonexistent. The main thing though is to intervene before things become too bad. In those cases, more extreme measures may be necessary. Understand what inflammatory disease is, recognize the signs and symptoms, and seek help when needed. Next, we will be discussing diet and its relationship to inflammation.

Chapter 2: Resolving Anti-Inflammatory Disease

We have spoken extensively about the inflammatory disease. It is important to shine a light on chronic inflammation in order to truly highlight the risks associated with the illness. To fix something, you must first understand what it is. Now that we have gone over the disease in-depth, we will start getting to the heart of this eBook. The main reason why we are here is to talk extensively about a major lifestyle change that can create very positive results. We are referring to the anti-inflammatory diet. You may have heard about this diet before. However, if you have not, we are here to tell you more about it. An important thing to remember is that each person's body is different. A strong consideration to make when altering your diet and overall lifestyle. Do your research and understand yourself. Assess thoroughly whether or not something is working well for you, especially based on how it makes you feel. This may not be conclusive, but a strong indicator of the benefits of something. Don't be afraid to speak up if you don't feel right. Don't be afraid to ask for help.

Anti-Inflammatory Diet

Mild inflammation is a necessary process for the body to protect itself. But prolonged and misguided inflammation is when things get out of hand. How can we resolve chronic inflammation or inflammatory disease? There are many ways. For this book, we will be focusing on the anti-inflammatory diet. Furthermore, we will focus specifically on vegan and vegetarian foods. These are really the meat, pardon the pun, of the diet as a whole. The vegetarian diet really encompasses more than we may think. There are actually different levels of vegetarianism and we hope to stay within those lines. Let's get started.

Let's begin with a couple of stories, shall we? Yes! More amazing stories. Just bear with us.

"Tommy is dealing with painful arthritis. He has been for a few months now and things are getting worse instead of better. It started in his hands but is now traveling to his neck and back. Also, it is becoming more difficult to walk long distances. Tommy eats a steady diet of cheeseburgers, pizza, fries, chocolate cakes, and sodas. This is what he likes, and this is what he eats. It is so delicious, so why would he stop? He heard about the anti-inflammatory diet, but he was not interested. He did not care for what this diet had to offer. Trading in burgers, pizza, and fries for whole grains, fish, fruits, and vegetables was not that appealing to him. He was a meat-eater through and through and he was not planning to change anytime soon. He wanted all of the fat, cholesterol, and sugar-filled foods. He kept eating and eating, until one day, he developed extreme chest pain. It was excruciating to the point he could not breathe. His feet were also starting to swell. He was sent to the hospital via emergency ambulance and is now diagnosed with heart disease and is also developing a digestive tract illness called Crohn's disease. The staff was also concerned about his labs that were showing early stages of kidney disease. The doctor informed him about the inflammation that had been going on for a very long time at this point. The chronic condition leads to more severe health consequences and Tommy will now need more aggressive therapies for his various ailments. Tommy is a busy guy running his business, taking care of his family, and needing to travel on a regular basis. Now, he is incapacitated to a degree with these various illnesses. He will have to start taking several different medications for blood pressure, cholesterol, pain, and diuretics to help excrete excess fluid. He will also have to make serious lifestyle changes immediately or things will continue to spiral out of control. He was literally weeks away from having a heart attack or something much worse. The damage has been done, but with a little help, things can still improve tremendously."

There's a strong chance that if Tommy would have listened to the warning signs earlier, he would need less drastic interventions. There were definitely plenty of warning signs. He either did not recognize them or did not care. Let's talk about what they were. The chronic pain was becoming worse and having difficulty walking long distances. These were some early signs that something was wrong. If the inflammation was affecting him outwardly like this, imagine what it may have been doing to him internally. Those whole grains and vegetables probably seem a lot more appealing than before.

Now, Tommy will need to take many medications and receive extensive therapies. Would an improved diet have fixed all of his problems? It is hard to say. There is no way of predicting this. The chances are, things would not have become as extreme as they did. You can run a red light, and nothing bad may happen. However, the chances of something bad happening increase dramatically. Same thing with our health. We can do everything right, and things can still go wrong. The chances of things going wrong though decrease dramatically if we do things right. Hopefully, Tommy can get his health together and make the necessary improvements in his life. Lucky for him, he was rushed to the hospital when he was. Things could have still turned out much worse for him. Let's talk about another story.

"Bobby loved eating high salt, high fat, and high sugary foods. His favorite thing to do was grease his eggs with a lot of extra butter. A few extra pieces of bacon on the side, plus some cut up and mixed into his eggs would usually suffice. He also loved a good chocolate muffin and a cup of coffee filled with creamer. His late-night snacks would consist of a slice of four-cheese pizza and pieces of salami. Burgers, pizza, fries, chicken, whatever was greasy was good for him and he would indulge whenever he could. A good lunch spot would be whatever fast-food restaurant he saw first. This was Bobby's daily life and he loved every moment of it. At some point, he began having neck pain. He figured this was normal due to the stress of is work. He had a pretty busy career with much responsibility. However, he began experiencing more muscle stiffness, fatigue, and soreness at the joints. His weight gain was increasing by the week as well. He decided he would go see his doctor. After getting a full checkup, Bobby's doctor informed him that he has some mild inflammatory disease. A combination of his diet and lifestyle were starting to weigh heavy on him. Lucky for him, it was still in the mild stages. He was still a young man in his thirties, but if he did not change things fast, he would be lucky to make it into the next decade.

Bobby still had a lot of living to do, so he made some life-altering changes. The most important one was his diet. He would still eat eggs every morning, but he cut down heavily on the butter. After a little while, he used none at all. He cut out the muffin and bacon and substituted some whole wheat toast. He drank his coffee black with half a teaspoon of sugar. He still liked his coffee a little sweet. For lunch, instead of getting a burger at a fast-food place, he would eat various fruits and salads, combined with various plant-based proteins for extra nutrition. Most of the time, he would make something healthy at home, like a sandwich made with whole wheat bread and take it with him. For a late-night snack, Bobby would eat an apple or avocado. He would indulge occasionally, but it was rare. This change in diet was not easy, but after a couple of weeks, when Bobby felt like a new person, he realized that it was totally worth it. When Bobby went in for his checkup the following month, his doctor was very satisfied. He had lost 10 pounds, his mobility had increased tremendously, and his lab results were impeccable. His energy levels throughout the day allowed him to be much more productive at work and in life. He still had a little way to do, but his progress so far had been remarkable. Eating all of those fat-filled foods may have brought some quick satisfaction, but the long-term effects were not worth it. In fact, the satisfaction of unhealthy foods was short-lived. The satisfaction of eating healthy, lasted all day. Especially since he was not feeling run down and exhausted. Most importantly, the timing was crucial. Lucky for him, he came in and got checked early, avoiding more serious health risks in the future. Bobby continues his new diet and is as happy as ever."

As you can see, Tommy and Bobby were heading down similar paths. Tommy ignored the warning signs, but Bobby didn't. Now, they are on two completely different roads. These two stories illustrate just how serious Inflammatory disease can be, and if caught early, can save you a world of trouble down the line. It can even save your life. Don't wait until you need more aggressive treatment like medications or surgery. If you are concerned, follow up with a healthcare provider and make the necessary changes as soon as you can. The anti-inflammatory diet can be a miracle when dealing with early stages of inflammatory disease. It takes work, it takes commitment, and it takes some sacrifice. But if you don't do it, you are sacrificing the worst thing you can; your health.

The anti-inflammatory diet is essentially an eating plan that is designed to prevent or reduce low-grade chronic inflammation. The key term is low-grade. That is why it is important to start early. The foods we ingest have a high level of influence on the amount of inflammation we experience, so sticking to an anti-inflammatory diet is essential to help avoid, resolve, or reduce chronic inflammation. While more extreme and invasive measures are available and may need to be taken with more severe cases; if something as simple as eating properly can avoid serious pain and health consequences, why not try it? Trading that greasy cheeseburger for a fresh salad may mean the difference between a healthy heart or a heart attack later on.

There is some controversy in the vegetarian world about exactly where the line is drawn. Veganism is considered the most extreme version of vegetarianism. However, some advocates will include poultry, fish, and dairy products as part of the vegetarian diet. Others will say no living creatures period. Some very devout vegetarians, like vegans, will even say no animal products period. We are not here to resolve this debate. However, we want to be respectful to those who embrace the vegetarian/vegan diet. Since there is a strong consensus that fish and dairy products are part of the diet or at least less extreme versions of it, we will include some fish and dairy products in our discussions, especially since so many of these foods are a strong addition to the anti-inflammatory diet. This is definitely true of oily fishes. Of course, if you leave these foods out, you can still combat inflammatory disease and get the proper nutrients. So, don't worry if you are a vegetarian and you don't want to include these certain foods. We have your back.

In a nutshell, an anti-inflammatory diet consists of foods that help to reduce or resolve the inflammation process. In fact, they are foods that most nutrition experts would encourage you to eat anyways. Fruits, vegetables, plant-based proteins, whole grains, nuts, beans, and fresh herbs and spices are all good food groups to turn to when going down this avenue. Most of these foods have compounds, like Omega-6 fatty acids, antioxidants, and polyphenols which have naturally occurring anti-inflammatory properties. Yes, this does limit the amount of food we can indulge, however, there is still a large variety of food we can choose from within these different food groups. There is a whole world of culinary goodness that will become open to you if you give it a chance and explore. Not only that, you will not feel awful after eating them. Eating should never make you feel worse than you already were. We will discuss various foods in more detail later in this chapter. For now, remember that the anti-inflammatory diet is not a cure-all plan. However, it can help us make significant steps in the right direction. Eat right and feel right: that is our motto for today.

Benefits of the Diet

With the anti-inflammatory diet, there have shown to be multiple benefits for a score of different diseases. One of the biggest being heart disease. Several studies have shown that an anti-inflammatory diet has reduced the risk of atherosclerosis in the arteries. As well, reduction in blood pressure, blood sugar, cholesterol levels, and obesity have been a common result of the anti-inflammatory diet. It makes sense, as the anti-inflammatory diet steers us away from all of the foods that consist of dangerous fats, excess cholesterol, and high sugar contents. As we mentioned earlier, the anti-inflammatory diet plays a significant role in reducing inflammation, which, in turn, reduces the risks of more severe health risks. Many prescribed diets in the hospital, such as the cardiac (heart) diet, diabetic diet, and the renal (kidney) diet resemble the anti-inflammatory diet in many ways while still having their own uniqueness. For example, the kidney diet discourages eating too many beans due to their high phosphorus content and also foods like tomatoes or bananas due to their potassium levels. With the anti-inflammatory diet, all of these are still okay. Therefore, once again, it's important to check with a professional before starting a life-altering diet plan. We want to make sure the diet has its intended purpose without shortchanging us on the nutrients we need to function. The cost of good health is nothing compared to the cost of poor health. Healthier ingredients may cost more at the beginning but can spare you big time in the long run.

Our sincere hope is that if you follow this diet, it will be a nutrient-rich lifestyle change and not just a short-lived experiment. If it's just for that, don't even bother because the results could be even more exhausting. Following this diet is not a quick fix. It takes work, sacrifice, and commitment. If you don't make the proper lifestyle changes, you may need some quick fixes to save your life. In the end, when you wake up feeling energized and ready to take on the day, you will realize that the hard work was worth it. Nothing good ever comes easy.

Different types of food that are part of the Anti-Inflammatory Diet

Now, let's get into the specifics about the foods that are part of the anti-inflammatory diet. While eating the diet may limit certain ingredients, we hope that it won't limit enjoyment. In fact, if given some time, we are certain that it won't. The various food groups, as well as the herbs and spices, can be combined in all sorts of fashion to create delicious meals. Also, it certainly will not limit nutrients. In this section, we will discuss various foods that are present inside of the different food groups that follow the anti-inflammatory diet plan.

- Whole grains - Whole grains, such as whole-oats, whole-wheat bread, brown rice, oatmeal, and Quinoa. Do not confuse whole grains with refined grains as refined grains are more processed, and thus not as nutritious. Whole grains keep all portions of the grain intact, which provide all of its nutrition and health benefits. Stick to the whole grains and you will stick to the diet. Don't worry, you don't have to eat grass, hay, or pure wheat. There are actually some delicious options here. Have you ever tried raw honey with fresh oatmeal? Maybe add a few berries on top? Yummy! Speaking of berries…

- Fruits - Some of the best anti-inflammatory foods include apples, cherries, berries (blueberries, raspberries, blackberries, and strawberries), oranges, grapes, and avocados. Many of the colorful compounds in the fruit have strong anti-inflammatory properties. Ever heard the term that an apple a day keeps the doctor away? This phrase is truer than we would like to admit. Of course, eating an apple a day may keep the doctor away, but if you don't go in for regular checkups, you're bananas. First the stories, now the jokes. We are on a roll here. Include these high-quality fruits in your daily diet. Since there are so many different kinds, it is easy to change things up every day. Eat an apple one morning, a banana the next, and then some blueberries the next. Trading in that chocolate candy bar for an apple or banana is a smart move in the long run. Wait, did we mention chocolates?

- Dark chocolate has been shown to exhibit some anti-inflammatory properties. Having it on occasion can still keep you on the anti-inflammatory diet route. Choose the chocolate that has a high percentage of cocoa. These will have flavonols which are another compound that will help reduce inflammation.

- Vegetables - Leafy green vegetables like kale, spinach, and collards have great anti-inflammatory properties. In addition, vegetables like broccoli, brussels sprouts, and cauliflower have anti-inflammatory effects due to their antioxidant properties. A good hearty salad can go a long way in making us feel good and satisfied. Be careful though, because many people will drown their salads with a lot of processed and unhealthy dressings. Don't worry though, there are healthier options if you just give them a chance. For example, squeezing pure lemon or lime can be beneficial and enhance the taste. If you are looking for a good dressing though, check out avocado dressing or cashew dressing. Both are great options that will satisfy the anti-inflammatory diet rules. Always double check salt content though. Salt can be hidden at times, and a silent killer. Vegetables, in general, are an important part of a wholesome diet. Fresh vegetables are very nutritive.

- Nuts - These include walnuts, almonds, pecans, and hazelnuts. Obviously, a handful of any of these is not going to satisfy anyone's cravings or make them full. However, various types of nuts can be added to foods, such as salads. Also, they can be used as a delicious snack, instead of a candy bar or chips. Various nuts, in general, have good types of fats that promote anti-inflammation. Make sure they are not processed kinds that are full of salt. Fresh nuts from your local grocery store or health food store will do. Roasting many of these different nuts can also enhance the taste. Keep some on hand with you and they will be a satisfying quick snack when you need it.

- Plants-based Proteins - These include chia seeds, soy products, almonds, quinoa, Tofu, edamame, peanuts, beans, potatoes, kale, chickpeas, and lentils. People's biggest concern about not eating meat is where they will get their protein.

However, there is a significant amount of protein in various vegetarian foods, and these proteins often create fewer chances of cardiovascular disease. Animal proteins will give you complete proteins with all amino acids but eating a variety of different plant-based proteins will do the same. Plus, things like quinoa and soybeans will also give you complete proteins. Think about some of the most powerful animals in the animal kingdom. Many of them have a vegetarian style diet. If it works for them, it can certainly work for us. "I feel as strong as a horse!" Some people will say. Well, horses are not chowing down on greasy hamburgers, that's for sure. Their eating some good old fashion hay.

- Oily Fishes - Oily fishes like salmon, trout, mackerel, tuna, and sardines are oily fishes that are good for fighting inflammation. Many still consider this part of the vegetarian diet, too, so we included them here. You can certainly leave these out if you choose to. However, they do have many health benefits and anti-inflammatory properties.

- Coffee - Several studies from top universities have shown that coffee and caffeine, in general, have strong anti-inflammatory properties. Coffee contains an anti-inflammatory compound called polyphenols, which help to defend against chronic inflammation. A morning cup of coffee may do just more than helps to wake you up. Remember not to go overboard. Watch that creamer and sweetener too. We are talking about black coffee here, not those crazy fancy drinks filled with sugar.

In general, foods that are rich in antioxidants, like many of the ones mentioned above, have strong anti-inflammatory properties as well. Furthermore, foods rich in Omega-3 fatty acids, also mentioned above, are also a strong addition to the anti-inflammatory diet. Much of the food we eat is rich in Omega-3 fatty acids as Omega-3 deficiency is very rare in the United States at least. Some examples of these foods include oily fish (salmon, mackerel, sardine, and anchovies), flaxseeds, chia seeds, soybeans, plant oils, eggs, and milk. One of the most heralded anti-inflammatory diets is the Mediterranean diet. We will discuss this in more detail later in this eBook when we get to the travel section. We have some delicious foods to talk about so don't go anywhere.

Other food options are tomatoes, green peppers, herbs and spices like garlic, cinnamon, rosemary, cloves, black pepper, ginger and turmeric, and sweet potatoes. It is advised to not use vegetable oils for cooking, but rather olive oil, soybean oil, or avocado oil. As you can see, the anti-inflammatory diet is largely vegan or vegetarian anyway. A big concern for many is that these types of diets lack many essential nutrients. This is a very legitimate concern. However, the anti-inflammatory diet is very well diverse and provides high levels of nutrition that our bodies need. We discussed proteins earlier, which is one of the more concerning nutrients we worry about lacking.

In further chapters, we will delve into more delicious meal plan options that will excite your palates. For now, many of these foods should satisfy your cravings and provide you the nutrition you need. While it is okay to indulge occasionally, it is important to remember that a healthy diet is good for your health and well-being as well as giving you a good quality of life. When you feel better, you live better. Imagine waking up in the morning and not feeling weak, not feeling bloated, not feeling pain, and not feeling ill. A proper anti-inflammatory diet will help put you on the right track to a well-balanced life.

While we have promoted these foods as a way to reduce inflammation when you have it, it is far better to prevent an issue than fix it later. Imagine if you incorporated these foods into your diet, even if you do not have an anti-inflammatory disease. This can majorly reduce the chances of having it in the first place and avoid major health concerns later in the future. Don't pick poor lifestyle choices simply because they are not affecting you now. They may have negative effects in the future. They could be doing untold damage that you do not even realize. It is easier to prevent than to fix. Remember, many of these diseases are silent killers. Meaning they won't present themselves until it is too late.

Foods to avoid

Food is an important part of our lives. It brings us happiness; it gives us memories; it gives us experiences. Food is essential and we should do our best to enjoy it to the fullest. Since we have discussed foods that you should incorporate into your diet to help reduce or prevent inflammation, we will also briefly touch on the foods to avoid. Diet obviously plays a huge role in our overall health. Much of our diet consists of fatty, high cholesterol, and high sugary foods, so they are very hard to avoid. Many foods that disguise themselves as healthy are anything but that. Unfortunately, many companies have hijacked the health food market and it is very difficult to distinguish the good from the bad. In general, these types of food should be balanced with the more healthy, anti-inflammatory options. The following is a list of some of the top foods and nutrients to avoid, especially if inflammation is already present.

- Foods rich in Omega-6 fatty acids are known to increase the body's production of inflammatory chemicals. These fatty acids do provide many other nutritional benefits that are necessary for us, so do not cut them out completely. Just balance them with the Omega-3 fatty acids we spoke about earlier and other foods associated with the anti-inflammatory diet. Some foods that are rich in Omega-6 fatty acids are red meats (burgers and steaks), French fries, and other fried foods and margarine. The jury is still out in a lot of ways on dairy products and whether they are good at fighting or increasing inflammation. It seems to vary based on the product itself. Dairy like yogurt seems to have positive anti-inflammatory effects, while things with a more fat content like cheese and whole milk have a negative effect. The benefits of milk can also be determined by how it's made. Besides yogurt, not much is known about other dairy products and their relationship to inflammation. Even many nutritional experts have a hard time understanding it. As a short, if they don't make you feel good, don't use them.

- Sodas and other sugary drinks should be avoided at all costs. They bring little to no nutritional value. While many of the foods we eat and beverages we drink have both positive and negative results, there really is no benefit to soda. A cool sparkling drink may taste good on a hot day, but there are other options to quench your thirst. Not only that, sodas only quench your thirst for a short period of time. Plus, they can cause you to excrete more fluid too, resulting in further dehydration. Avoid sodas for a healthier option and be careful when choosing those healthier options.

- Sweets like cakes and cookies. It can be tempting to order that large piece of cake after a large meal but try to avoid it if you can. Food filled with high sugar content is one of the worst things for inflammation, especially considering the portion sizes we have today. Eating refined carbohydrates can have similar results.

- Coffee creamers and anything else with trans-fat which raise LDL levels, leading to inflammation. Enjoy that cup of coffee, black, without the creamer. Other foods high in trans-fat include doughnut, snack foods like microwave popcorn, frozen foods, fast-food, and ready to use frostings. It is better to stick with natural foods than processed foods as a rule of thumb.

- Refined carbs like white bread, white rice, pastries, white pasta, breakfast cereals, and refined grains can increase inflammation. Stick to the whole grains which are more nutrient-rich at better at fighting inflammation. Have a bowl of oatmeal instead of that sugary cereal in the morning. If you're having toast, stick to whole wheat bread instead of white bread. Enjoy the pasta, but make it whole wheat pasta.

- Avoid processed vegetable oils. Plant-based oils are recommended.

Most of these are probably foods that you have been told all your life to either avoid or limit. All the great stuff that we love, right? In actuality, many of the foods we mentioned in the previous section can be healthy and delicious, or even combined to create delicious foods. While you don't have to cut out all the food we discussed in this section completely, it is important to limit and balance with a healthy and nutritious diet.

As with any diet or major lifestyle change, it is important you do it in a safe and nondetrimental manner. It is advised to consult a healthcare provider or nutrition expert when drastically changing diet plans. While it's good to switch to more nutritious options, we also want to make sure we don't exclude necessary nutrients. We will be driving this point home constantly like it's a broken record. Records? What are those? Look it up, please.

Chapter 3: History of the Anti-Inflammatory Diet

To better understand the significance of the anti-inflammatory diet, it is important to research the history and fundamentals behind it. In doing this, we can shine a better light on the whole phenomenon. As you will see, it is not a new fad that just gained popularity out of nowhere. A bunch of celebrities did not just start promoting it and now suddenly, it has taken over the world. Never do something just because it is popular. That being said, this particular diet has been popular for a long time. The diet predates modern times and modern medicine. We will touch on the history here so we can better understand the fundamentals. Understanding our history makes it easier to understand our present.

The origins of the anti-inflammatory diet date back to some of the original healers in the world and throughout history. Many of these healers worked with natural herbs, foods, teas, and other holistic remedies to assist the body with its own healing process. Much of these practices are still performed by various people around the world. Without having access to modern, manufactured medications, these natural healers had to make do with what they had. What they did have was an abundance of natural ingredients at their disposal to use for healing or preventing certain ailments. While there may not have been a lot of scientific research to back up many of their claims, much anecdotal evidence suggested that they were on to something. Much of what people discover of the past helped people learn more during the present. While the advent of modern medicines should be held up with pride, it is important to give credit to natural remedies that helped heal people for centuries. Much of it was related to the food people ate.

In more modern times, the anti-inflammatory diet really began getting more mainstream attention from the medical community in the 1970s. Around this time, researchers found that naturally occurring proteins found in our body were a major cause of tissue injury. Before this time, it was believed to be pathogens from outside of the body. This new finding of substances in our own body damaging our own tissues was a big breakthrough for the researchers of this time. They began realizing that our own bodies cells can do just as much, if not more damage than outside sources. Our body literally has the ability to destroy itself. Remember earlier how we spoke of misguided inflammation? This is essentially substances in our own body attacking itself and its own internal tissues, like these proteins, were discovered to do. This was a huge breakthrough for the medical sciences and the makings of an anti-inflammatory diet. Once they discovered this breakthrough, they could better understand how to fix it.

Then in the 1980s, further evidence suggested that various proteins in our bodies were either beneficial or injurious to our bodies' tissues. One of the newly named proteins of this time were called cytokines, which were produced by the immune system. The release of these proteins during the inflammatory process was seen to cause damaging results after the effects of chronic disease. Researchers also began using C-reactive protein, which is a marker of inflammation circulating the blood as a way to identify persons at risk of chronic disease.

More advanced research found that people with higher levels of C-reactive proteins also had higher levels of heart disease. With much of the research indicating these results, a growing consensus to this day is that inflammation plays a very significant role in the pathogenesis of chronic illnesses like heart disease, lung disease, stroke, diabetes, kidney disease, and even some cancers. For this reason, many medical practitioners and nutrition experts are promoting certain anti-inflammatory diets with foods that will reduce the amount of inflammation in our bodies. This reduced inflammation will result in decreasing or even preventing more chronic illnesses. The anti-inflammatory diet is becoming more prominent as the push to prevent illness rather than cure it is taking off. People are realizing once more that it is better to prevent a catastrophe than deal with its aftermath. The promotion of a proper anti-inflammatory diet coupled with other major lifestyle changes can work wonders for aiding in chronic illnesses.

While we will never discredit the advances of modern medicine, we also want to pay homage to the healers and practitioners of the past. Without the work they did, we would not have made the modern-day strides to continue and advance health and medicine. We also cannot deny that techniques of the past were essential in improving health and we certainly should not avoid these practitioners' contributions for what we have today. Without there knowledge and discoveries, we could not have advanced as much as we have. If it worked for them in the past, then it can work for us today. Modern medicine is needed to deal with some of the advanced medical problems we have today. However, with proper diet and lifestyle, we can prevent those problems from occurring in the first place. Both theories and practices can coexist.

Ancient Greek physician, Hippocrates, who is often considered the Father of Medicine, was one of the first to understand the impact of environment, diet, and lifestyle on human health. Before this, people just related it to external sources like Gods or demons. Hippocrates approach to medicine is far removed from today's medical practices. Modern-day medicine is believed to take a more curative and diagnostic approach, while with Hippocrates, it was focused more on patients care and a good prognosis. Basically, preventative care. Both schools of thought existed in Hippocrates' day, the other one sharing more similarities with the medical practices of today.

Even though much of Hippocrates principles are outdated in ways, his approach can still be heralded as well. With the advent of advanced techniques, we can cure illnesses that were death sentences in years past. It is amazing how far we have come with medical science and we will continue to do so as the years go by. However, our focus with the anti-inflammatory diet somewhat plays off of the teachings of Hippocrates and his beliefs of lifestyle, environment, and diet impacting our health. While at times, extreme measures and advanced medicine is needed, to deny something like diet and lifestyle not having an effect on health is irresponsible.

Let's consider this for a second: remember our two stories from earlier about Tommy and Bobby? Tommy did not use preventative approaches to fix his health. Now, he needs to rely on more advanced medicine to fix his ailments. We applaud the fact that these advanced techniques are available to save Tommy's life. However, we also acknowledge that if Tommy made several lifestyle changes earlier, he may not have needed these more aggressive therapies. With Bobby, he made the changes in his diet early, and for that reason, his health is much better off. We contend that it is better to prevent a heart attack than cure one after the fact.

In summary, the diet in some form has existed for centuries around the world. With further research and determination of the pathogenesis of several diseases, the benefits of the diet's effect on chronic illness are undeniable. We realize that we went more in-depth than we needed to in discussing the science behind inflammatory disease. However, understanding the illness gives us a better understanding of the cure. The anti-inflammatory diet exists also in various forms around the world and we will discuss this further when we get into traveling with the anti-inflammatory diet. There is no one-size-fits-all plan when it comes to this diet and that is what makes it great. Anyone can find food that they love within the parameters of the diet.

Chapter 4: The Diet and You

Now that we have discussed the diet extensively, let's put it all together. We will bring it full circle and discuss how the diet can and will affect you. It will impact you in a big way, especially, if you are used to eating a lot of meat, high saturated fat, high sugar, and high cholesterol foods. The anti-inflammatory diet pretty much eliminates all of that. Also, a common routine we have been taught is to have three large meals at breakfast, lunch, and dinner. With the anti-inflammatory diet, it is suggested to have five or six smaller meals throughout the day. Eating multiple times throughout the day keeps up your metabolism and decreases the major fluctuations in blood sugar that come from eating fewer and larger meals. This is easier on your internal organs, especially your pancreas.

The diet alone is not a cure-all. It should be coupled with a healthy lifestyle in general. There are much literature and information out there about living healthy in many ways. For this Book, we will still focus on the diet more than anything else. The first thing you should do is identify the signs or symptoms that may be concerning to you. Whether you feel healthy or not, regular checkups are very important. With the assistance of a professional, begin eliminating certain unhealthy foods from your diet and start incorporating more foods related to an anti-inflammatory diet. Do this whether you are dealing with inflammation or not. For example, eat fewer red meats and poultry and start eating more oily fishes, beans, lentils, soy, and tofu for protein. Furthermore, replace your unhealthy sugary snacks with healthier options like fruits. Also, for meals, eat vegetable, whole grains, and various nuts for snacks. Having foods like this throughout various times of the day will increase energy, concentration, and help you avoid more long-term illnesses. Prepare foods the night before so you have it with you for the next day. This limits the number of times you have to eat out. Diet and how it affects us is truly a science, so that is why it is important to consult a professional.

It is best to also eat around the same times every day. This can be quite difficult with the busy lives that we live, but with some extra effort, it can be done. Carry small, healthy snacks like almonds or apples with you. Allowing you to eat at a moment's notice. Set aside a certain amount of time throughout the day to sit and eat. Eat a good meal before you start your day. Incorporate your eating habits into your everyday life and make them a priority. Making your dietary selections a priority is not really an option if you want a healthy and more fulfilling life. It is a necessity. Write things down, and you will remember them better. You will also start holding yourself accountable.

This chapter was written with the assumption that you are currently not following the anti-inflammatory diet whatsoever. For this reason, we gave you some of the most fundamental techniques to help integrate the diet into your lifestyle. We apologize if it may come off as judgmental, but we sincerely hope this will help you in your daily routine. We will talk more about setting up a schedule further in this book. For now, think about ways you can replace certain unhealthy foods for more nutritious options. Replace that sugary coffee with black coffee or green tea. Replace that lunchtime burger for a fresh salad. Replace that greasy pasta dinner for some whole wheat pasta. Finally, replace that late-night sugary snack for an avocado or banana. Enjoy the results of this new lifestyle.

Let's tell another short story. Oh, come on! Another one? Yes, they're not so bad, are they? This will just be a short day in the life of someone starting an anti-inflammatory diet. Let's call it… A Day in The Life of Someone Starting an Anti-Inflammatory Diet. We'll call our person Amanda.

Amanda is planning to start a new life. After living with many health problems, she has decided to turn a new leaf and start a new diet that was directed by her doctor. It is Saturday night and she plans to start her new diet, the anti-inflammatory diet, the following morning. This is in relation to her chronic inflammation caused by some auto-immune disorder. Her current diet and lifestyle are not compatible with the disease, so she has to make some changes. And she is willing to. After a fun night out with her friends, she goes back home and retires for the night. She is excited and ready to start her new lifestyle. She is also a little nervous, too. This will definitely be a big change for her, and she will have to give up a lot of the foods she loves and is used to. She can do it though.

The next morning, it is Sunday and things are about to change. Amanda looks in her refrigerator and sees nothing but junk food. She has to fix this. She looks at her countertop and sees nothing but sugary foods. This is another thing that has to change. Amanda decides she has to go to the store and pick up a few things. But what will she eat for breakfast? Normally, she would have some type of toaster pastry or chocolate muffin and chase it down with orange juice or chocolate milk. She knew she could not do this today. She cannot start her new day by repeating the mistakes of the past. But she was not sure what choice she would have. She looked in her fridge a little bit more and saw that she has some eggs. She figures this is the best thing for her. She starts breaking them apart and mixing them. As she is getting the pan ready, she realizes that she usually coats it with butter. She decides not to do that today. She continues to make the eggs. She also prepares a cup of coffee. Normally, she adds a lot of French vanilla creamer. On this morning, she still adds a little bit, but just half the amount as before. She also adds just one spoon of sugar versus two. A few small steps in the right direction. She may not be able to make all of the drastic changes at once. It's ok though, it will be a slightly slow transition as long as she realizes she has to make the changes soon.

After Amanda is done eating her breakfast, she heads to the store. She has a list of various food products given to her by her doctor and dietician in order to stick to the anti-inflammatory diet. She walks down the various aisles and picks out a few things. She avoids buying any red meats for now. She picks up some tofu and salmon instead. For snacks, she gets some almonds, peanuts, walnuts, and cashews. She also gets some carrot sticks and celery. While walking by the candy aisle, she looks but keeps moving. She moves to the dairy products and picks up some Greek yogurt and some more eggs. She refuses to get more butter. The last thing she gets are some lentils, broth for her soups, and various types of beans, including kidney beans and garbanzo beans. Her last stop before checking out is the fruits' section. She picks up some apples, bananas, blueberries, raspberries, oranges, and avocados. As she is walking up to the register, she sees that she has foods from most of the major groups.

While standing at the register, she notices the candy bars at the checkout stand again. She tries to resist but then picks one up. It is one of her guilty pleasures. Well, she won't get rid of all of her bad habits in one day. After all, she has already made a lot of progress already. She is making a lot of the right decision. After leaving the stores, she realizes that she has a lot of cooking to do. It will probably take her the rest of the day as she does not have many nutritious items at her home. As she is driving, she notices a Mediterranean restaurant, which she heard is some of the healthiest food around, so she stops in. She buys a falafel salad and pita bread with hummus. All pretty healthy food that will fill her up for most of the day. She takes her food and starts driving home, excited about trying something new.

When Amanda arrives home, she starts eating her food so that she can begin cooking. She really enjoys the falafel, which is a patty made from chickpeas. It is a very wholesome and delicious protein option. That mixed with the salad is really tasty for her. She cannot finish all of the pita bread and hummus, so she will save it for later. The food really filled her up and she was excited to try a variety of other foods after this, especially, international foods which also follow the anti-inflammatory diet plan in many ways.

She slowly gets up from the table and starts putting things away. The first thing she realizes is that she has to clear her fridge of all of the junk she had in it before. This will take her a few minutes. She felt bad about getting rid of so much of her favorite food, but it was for her health. After getting rid of the old food, she stocked her fridge and cabinets with the newer items. She was truly making a lifestyle change for the better. From now on, she would do her best to stick with a vegetarian anti-inflammatory diet. It would be tough, she knew this, but it would be worth it. The fact that she liked the falafel salad gave her inspiration to try new food.

After everything was put away, Amanda began cooking. With all of the ingredients she bought, she began cooking up some new meals that she never tried before. She was mixing the various beans that she bought with the various spices. Not really knowing what she was doing but still willing to put in the effort. It would be interesting how this would all play into her new life. As Amanda stirred the pot, she was ready to begin the next phase. She was ready for life on the anti-inflammatory diet.

This is Amanda's story. Maybe it will be similar to yours. Whatever the case, start incorporating the anti-inflammatory diet into your life. It won't be easy, but it will be worth it. Later on, in this

Book, we will look at a more in-depth schedule surrounding the anti-inflammatory diet and how it can play a role in your life. You will be able to interact more so and put yourself into that story.

And if you need a reminder: Whole grains, fruits, vegetables, nuts, beans, plant-based proteins, and oily fishes (salmon, mackerel, tuna, etc.). Stick to these foods and you will stick to the anti-inflammatory diet.

Chapter 5: Tasty meals

We discussed previously the various foods and food groups that are part of the anti-inflammatory diet. Now, we will put it all together. We will discuss some specific recipes that are both nutritious and delicious. We mentioned before that you may have to sacrifice certain types of food, without sacrificing taste. Let's see if some of these recipes will tickle your fancy. Now, this is not a cookbook, so we will not be getting into measurements or cooking methods in anyways. There are plenty of cookbooks out there available for that. We will simply name some dishes and discuss how they fit into the anti-inflammatory diet. Once again, we are sticking to vegan and vegetarian foods. There is a lot of debate still whether or not things like fish and dairy products are part of a vegetarian diet. People who also eat fish and dairy products are considered a milder form of a vegetarian. Considering that certain fishes and dairy products are a major part of some anti-inflammatory diets, we have included them here. You can certainly leave those out and still have plenty of nutritious foods available to you. Some people even include poultry like chicken in the vegetarian diet because it is not meat. We do not include it here, sorry. We are dedicated to making the world love vegetarian food. We want you to love it also.

- Freshly grilled salmon is a very tasty and popular dish. Many types of fish, like salmon, have a high omega-3 fatty acid content, which helps to reduce certain inflammatory proteins, like C-reactive proteins, in our bodies. There are many ways to grill salmon and adding extra vegetable can make it even better.

- Next up, we have red beans with brown rice. Here we have a combination of beans and whole grains. Two powerful food groups that play a huge part in the anti-inflammatory process. Beans and whole grains have several anti-inflammatory agents and antioxidants. If you don't like kidney beans, try pinto beans, black beans, or garbanzo beans. There are several recipes out there to help you cook these various beans in a nutritious and tasty manner. It is interesting because you can get creative with your cooking. Make sure you are using brown rice. Avoid white rice.

- Sandwiches with whole grain wheat bread and some onions combined with other vegetables, like leafy greens, tomatoes, or avocados. Most of these vegetables and tomatoes have strong anti-inflammatory properties also. Sandwiches with a variety of different vegetables and whole grains are always a good option.

- Sweet potatoes without the salt, accompanied with black pepper, chives, and tomatoes. Avoid frying them in vegetable oil or you will lose the anti-inflammatory properties of sweet potatoes. In fact, bake it and don't fry it. And once again, cut out the salt. Salt is not our friend in this case.

- Arctic Char with Chinese Broccoli and Sweet Potato Puree. This dish is a combination of sweet potatoes, broccoli, balsamic vinegar, and Chinese mustard. You can substitute American mustard for Chinese mustard if needed. Once again, you can make these recipes your own.

- A nice regular baked potato without all of the fix-ins, especially without the sour cream. Remember that a baked potato is healthy, but when you start adding all of the sour cream, salt, and extra ingredients, not so much. It is better to just have French fries.

- A salad with spinach, kale, onions, garbanzo beans, and lettuce. A light salad that is healthy and will help fight inflammation. Can use a little olive oil dressing also. Perhaps even some lemon juice or a vinaigrette dressing.

- Smoked salmon salad with avocado dressing. This salad is loaded with salmon, which as we mentioned before, is filled with omega-3 fatty acid. Green lentils, spinach, red onions, parsley, and baby capers are also a part of this delicious salad. This is a filling meal that is rich in foods that help fight chronic inflammation. A very full meal rich with protein that would kick that red meat to the curb.

- Black Bean Salad with cashew dressing. Black beans, various spices and herbs like garlic, cumin and turmeric, red onions, zucchini, fresh corn, red chili, and coriander leaves. The cashew dressing is a combination of cashews, olive oil, lemon juice, and water. All of these foods are rich in antioxidants and anti-inflammatory agents. A combination of them together is the ultimate meal to fight chronic inflammation.

- Oat and Berry acai bowl. A combination of a purple fruit called acai, a mixture of different berries, chia seeds, milk, and bananas. A rich breakfast meal that fights inflammation. Many of the compounds in colorful fruits like acai are great for fighting inflammation.

- Whole grain oatmeal is another strong breakfast food that fits the anti-inflammatory diet. Add some blueberries, bananas, strawberries, apples, and many other fruits you desire. This is much more desirable than breakfast cereals.

- Roasted salmon with potatoes and romaine. A combination of fresh salmon, potatoes, romaine lettuce, lemon juice, and paprika cooked in olive oil.

- Grilled Avocado, hummus, and sauerkraut. All great options and a great combination for fighting inflammation. Again, give some of these foods a chance. They might surprise you.

- Buckwheat and chia seed porridge. Buckwheat is a great substitution for oats, especially for those who have gluten sensitivities. A very good whole grain. Chia seeds are a great source of Omega-3 fatty acids.

- Buckwheat berry pancakes are a great breakfast food. It has everything you need to tackle the inflammatory disease. A great addition to the anti-inflammatory diet.

- Smoked salmon, avocado, and poached eggs on whole-wheat toast. Or, how about a whole wheat bagel. A great option either way.

- Quinoa and Citrus salad-some of these foods speak for themselves and just scream anti-inflammatory diet. We can practically hear this one yelling through the computer right now.

- Lentils, beetroot, and hazelnut salad. An exciting combination of anti-inflammatory foods. A great addition to any meal, night or day. Lentils seem to be taking over the world day by day.

- Roasted Root Vegetables-Maple syrup and fall spices added to a combination of vegetables. Sweet potatoes, beets, parsnips, turnips, and extra virgin olive oil. This is a delectable fall treat, especially with the addition of the maple syrup.

- Steak! Got you excited, didn't I? Yes, you can have a delicious steak!!! It is wholesome and delicious. Our next recipe will excite the heck out of you. It is time for some cauliflower steak with beans and tomatoes. Yes, a wonderful vegan steak option that is full of anti-inflammatory foods. Cauliflower mixed with various herbs and spices combines with beans of your choice and tomatoes. The New York strip or filet minion has nothing on this bad boy. No, we are not being sarcastic! Give it a try. We think you may be impressed.

- Lettuce wraps with smoked trout. Trout is another fatty fish rich in Omega-3 fatty acids used to fight inflammation.

- Zucchini pasta with pesto. Zucchini pasta is a great alternative to regular pasta, especially for those with gluten sensitivities.

- Roasted cauliflower, fennel, and ginger soup are filled with anti-inflammatory compounds called polyphenols. Ginger adds some needed antioxidants.

- Lentil soup with sweet potatoes-Need we say more. This is a hearty soup and if you eat a bowl, it can be a meal, too. But just in case, eat some more sweet potatoes on the side. A great source of fiber and proteins. Great for a cold day while staying inside.

- Salmon with green vegetables and cauliflower - There goes that cauliflower again. Maybe you can add that steak we spoke about earlier to this meal. Brussels sprouts are a good addition to this meal, along with many other green vegetables.

- Vegetable curry with carrots, red peppers, and peas and two spoons of turmeric. Oops, maybe we should have put this in the international section instead. Oh well, curry is very popular around the world. Plus, we have already been getting a little international anyways. Don't worry though, there is more to come.

- Vegetarian Chili - Chili is a hearty meal to eat on a cold day. Or really, on any day for that matter. You can still enjoy a good bowl of chili while sticking to the anti-inflammatory diet. This can be a versatile dish filled with various types of beans and vegetables to your liking. Enjoy and make yourself a nice big bowl of vegetarian chili. Don't skimp on the beans and vegetables. A good combination would be kidney beans, red peppers, carrots, and onions.

- Whole wheat waffles with maple syrup, topped with blueberries and raspberries.

- Chickpea, cauliflower salad. Uses the cauliflower and chickpeas as the base, added on are lettuce, onions, and tomatoes. Very delightful salad to fight off inflammatory disease.

- A delicious salad mixed with red bell pepper, spinach, and goat cheese, topped with oregano dressing.

- Here is a good snack option: Chia seed pudding. A combination of chia seeds, coconut milk, maple syrup, pineapple, and raspberries. A great snack to indulge on for sure.

This is just the tip of the iceberg for anti-inflammatory recipes. We could write several types of cookbooks to include all of them. You can use the combination of various foods in so many ways in order to fit your palate. We just want to emphasize that meal options are not so limited when sticking to an anti-inflammatory diet. Coming up with all these various recipes is quite joyful. A great game you can make for yourself is to try and top what you make every day. See just how much of an anti-inflammatory meal you can make and judge which one of them would fight anti-inflammatory disease the most. Maybe, you can even hold a contest with your friends and give out prizes. This will get your friends involved in your healthy lifestyle as well. We want you to and encourage you to be as creative as possible. It is easier to do things with a team anyway. We know this is a lot to take in. Just remember though: Whole grains, fruits, vegetable, nuts, beans, plant-based proteins, and oily fishes. Stay on this route with the foods and you will do well. I just want to thank you for making it this far. It is amazing to be able to share these recipes with you and be an interactive part of your health and wellness. Keep reading for some great information.

Let's mention a few drinks, shall we:

- Green smoothies can be made in various ways. With much of the ingredients having anti-inflammatory effects. A popular recipe includes a combination of almond milk, bananas, mixed berries, flaxseed, and spinach.

- Green Tea has a rich source of a substance called polyphenol, which has been shown to reduce inflammation. Maybe, replace that coffee or Frappuccino in the morning for a nice cup of green tea.

- Coffee - A good cup of coffee is always nice. Coffee is known to have several anti-inflammatory properties. Brew some up today.

- Pineapple and ginger juice - Filled with celery stalks, cucumber, pineapple, apple, lemon, spinach, and ginger.

- Berry Beet Smoothie - Beets, oranges, strawberries, turmeric, and ginger. Filled with a lot of fruits as well as herbs and spices that fight inflammation.

- Pure pineapple juice has been shown to reduce pain, inflammation, and swelling. Often times, given to people who are recovering from surgery.

- Apple Cider Vinegar Drink - Apple cider vinegar, lemon, honey, and cayenne pepper. This is really good for an inflamed stomach.

- Pickle juice - This has been a miracle for so many people and their ailments.

- Pineapple smoothie - Now this just sounds plain delicious.

- Fresh juice made from kale, celery, ginger, apples, and lemons. What a great combination of some powerful fruits and vegetable to fight inflammation. This is a great dichotomy of sweet and salty.

- Beets juice mixed with carrots, apples, lemons, and ginger. The powerful taste of beets will likely overtake this juice. Beets are a wonderful vegetable for our health and work well to prevent inflammation in our bodies.

- A vegetable juice with spinach, celery, cucumbers, carrots, and kale. Another great combination of vegetables.

- Infused water with cucumber and lemons. A great infused drink that is refreshing and also healthy.

- Drink a glass of lemon water every morning with some raw honey and apple cider vinegar. You can also infuse some other fruits into the water, like oranges or kiwi.

Just like with food, get creative with your drinks. Take all of the various fruits and vegetables and make your own drinks from them. One day, have a carrot, apple, and pineapple juice. The next day, have blueberry, strawberry, and banana smoothie. It is advised to avoid the premade processed juices that you find at the store. These options are oftentimes no better than sodas. Try to make your own or at least find a juice place that makes them fresh every day. From now on, make certain commitments to yourself. Instead of reaching for a candy bar, reach for some almonds. Instead of grabbing a processed cheeseburger from a fast-food place, make a salad or eat some fresh salmon. Go to the Mediterranean restaurant and pick up some hummus. Go after fresh food and not quick food. Make more food at home instead of going out. If you are going out, go to a quality restaurant that serves fresh food. Make a commitment to yourself and to your health, because nobody else will.

There are many more recipes out there that are delicious and flavorful. You can combine the various food groups in so many ways in order to make appetizing meals. Get creative and make it an art form. Challenge yourself and see just how extreme you can get in making an anti-inflammatory meal. Now, we understand that if you are a heavy meat eater, these meals may sound disappointing at first, but give them a chance. Unfortunately, red meats do not fare well with this diet. Even so, we are sticking to vegan and vegetarian foods. A combination of these various foods and flavors will provide a rich, hearty meal that may even make you not miss any meat. They will also allow you to have the nutrients you will need that you think will be missing from a nonmeat diet. We hope that these meal plans have tickled your fancy a little bit and you will give the anti-inflammatory diet a chance. If for nothing else, your own health and well-being. We will get into more delicious foods when we start talking about traveling the world and enjoying the various culinary treats from around the globe. Trust us, there is much more to come.

Chapter 6: Traveling with the Anti-Inflammatory Diet

Sticking to a strict diet should not negatively affect your lifestyle. In fact, the whole purpose of discussing the anti-inflammatory diet is to help improve your overall lifestyle. Why do something if it will just make you miserable. We are confident that eating the variety of foods in the anti-inflammatory diet playbook will satisfy your cravings and your palate. Maybe not at first, but it will grow on you. We are sure of this. One of the most fun things about traveling is being able to enjoy the various foods we come across. These foods are delicious and offer so much variety. It is a great experience to walk around and partake in the various delicacies that exist. Unfortunately, many of these foods may not be the healthiest in their nature. Most of them may not even come close to following the anti-inflammatory diet. We would never want you to miss an opportunity to try some new food, especially, if it is something you won't get a chance to try again. So, definitely indulge a little bit, especially when you are traveling and having the time of your life. Remember though, to not go overboard, especially if you already have an inflammatory disease. The level at which you have inflammation also greatly affects when and how much you can indulge. Definitely take this into account. No amount of fun is worth risking your health like that. You know yourself better than anyone else. We do not want you to become severely ill when you are traveling. Nothing could put a bigger damper on your world tour than this. We don't want you to end up in a hospital bed when you should be seeing the sites.

That being said, we want you to be able to travel, enjoy healthy meals, and also get a taste of the distinct dishes without cheating on your diet. For this reason, we will discuss several culinary favorites from various regions around the world that will keep you devoted to the anti-inflammatory diet.

We will break this down place by place. We will continue with vegan and vegetarian options. We hope that we have done a good job with that so far, so we will keep going with this. The world is ours for the taking, so let's get to traveling and see where we end up.

Mediterranean:

Ok, we will begin right here. This seems to be the Mecca of the anti-inflammatory diets. This makes a lot of sense as the majority if not all, foods and food groups that are considered part of the anti-inflammatory diet are also in the Mediterranean diet. Mediterranean food has a lot of influence from Europe, Eastern Europe, and the Middle East based on its geographical location. Go to an authentic Mediterranean restaurant and you will see for yourself. A solid Mediterranean diet will give you energy and rarely ever make you feel bloated, ill, or tired. The diet and region incorporate so much great food that is quite delicious. The vegetarian foods in this diet are flavorful to the point that you will not be missing that steak or cheeseburger. At least not for a while. And remember, there is always that cauliflower steak. Here are some popular meals included in the diet. Again, this is not a cookbook, so we will not be discussing specific measurements or food prepping processes.

- Classic Greek Salad - A strong stable that is part of Mediterranean cuisine. A combination of cucumbers, tomatoes, olives, red onions, feta, and Greek dressing make for a delicious treat. A Mediterranean salad is quite filling, but not overbearing. A nice whole wheat pita bread on the side is a great addition. You can eat this as an appetizer, but it will probably work as a full meal too.

- Spicy Escarole with Garlic - Escarole is a leafy green, somewhat bitter vegetable. By itself, it may not be that appetizing, but combined with other ingredients, it can become a tasty treat. This meal is a combination of the leafy green vegetable with garlic, olive oil, and red pepper flakes. It is light. Can be used as an appetizer or main course, depending on how hungry you are. Whatever the case, a great addition to the anti-inflammatory diet.

- Eggplant with yogurt and dill - This is a common side dish of the region. Roasted eggplant, garlic, shallots, and walnuts tossed with yogurt and fresh dill. A shallot is a type of onion and onions are a great addition to the diet. You will see a lot of dishes with eggplant in the Mediterranean diet. A very powerful food in fighting inflammation. Help kick inflammatory disease to the burb.

- Broccoli Rabe with Cherry Peppers - Not to be confused with regular broccoli, broccoli rabe is a green leafy vegetable that is part of the turnip family. The edible parts are the leaves, bulbs, and stem. In this particular dish, the bitter vegetable is mellowed out by adding spicy cherry peppers, garlic, and some rich parmesan cheese.

- Cauliflower Couscous - Couscous tossed with sautéed cauliflower and shallots. Cinnamon and dates are added for natural sweetness. Cauliflower is a vegetable that is a strong addition to the anti-inflammatory diet. It is also big in the Mediterranean diet. Cinnamon is also a great spice to add to the anti-inflammatory diet.

- Tabbouleh - An herb lover's dream come true. This is a salad that usually has a bulgur base, however, other things like quinoa and rice. Whatever the base, it is mixed with fresh tomatoes, onions, parsley, mint, and a tangy lemon vinaigrette. People are often generous with the mint and parsley to make it fresher and more flavorful. Bulgur is a cereal food made from several different wheat spices. Tabbouleh can be eaten by itself or even with some pita bread.

- Pepper and Peanut Broccoli Stir-fry - Combination of red pepper, red chili flakes, Broccoli florets, and chopped, roasted, and unsalted peanuts.

- Bulgur Salad - Bulgur is a traditional whole grain. This salad is a combination of bulgur, cucumber olives, and dill.

- Falafel pita with lettuce, tomatoes, onions, and peppers. Falafel is a very popular protein in this type of diet, often replacing chicken or beef. It is a patty made from chickpeas. You can also have this as a delicious salad. What are you waiting for?

- Eggplant, lentils, and peppers cooked in olive oil. Yep, remember that olive oil or avocado oil.

- Baba Ghanoush - Mixed eggplant, tahini made from sesame seeds, olive oil, and various seasonings. A very popular appetizer of the region.

- You can also just enjoy a good snack like some hummus and pita bread, or a nice yogurt topped with berries.

- Greek yogurt with strawberries and oats.

- A tuna salad dressed in olive oil.

- Mediterranean Pizza. A delicious pizza without all of the healthy fat. It is topped with cheese, vegetables, and olive. The crust is made of whole wheat.

- Egg white omelet with veggies and olives.

- Yogurt with sliced fruits and nuts.

- Broiled Salmon served with brown rice and vegetables.

- If you want to add cheese, choose feta cheese.

- The drink of choice for sticking to a Mediterranean diet is good old-fashioned water. Avoid all of those sugary juices.

There are so many recipes in the Mediterranean diet that would kick inflammatory disease to the curb. Unfortunately, we cannot mention all of them, because that would take a whole other book. Actually, maybe several since the recipes are so abundant. Just know that if you're following the Mediterranean diet, you are probably on the right track. The best thing about the Mediterranean diet is that it is filling, but you will not feel heavy. You will probably never feel bloated. Great for the digestive tract. Your gut will be very happy with you. Mediterranean food consists of a strong combination of whole grains, fruits vegetables, beans, nuts, and various spices. It is indeed an anti-inflammatory diet eaters dream.

India:

If Mediterranean food is the ultimate anti-inflammatory diet, Indian food may just come in as a close second. Indian food often promotes a strongly vegetarian diet mixed with an abundance of herbs, spices, vegetables, beans, whole wheat, and lentils. The protein content is strong with Indian food. The food also promotes a high fiber diet, which has also been known to fight inflammation. Of course, Indian food is known for its spice level. Many people outside of the subcontinent can barely tolerate it. So, if you're asking someone to prepare you a dish, take this into account. While various spices can be very healthy for you, it does you no good if you can't eat it anyway. Take in the spices at your own risk and your own tolerance level. That being said, it will be difficult to find culinary options that are more flavorful than Indian food. Let's get our spice on.

- Before we start with specific meals, here are some herbs and spices that are powerful anti-inflammatories which are common in India: Bay leaves, black pepper, cardamom, and cloves. Along with some of their anti-inflammatory properties, these herbs and spices are used for a lot of ailments in general, like pain and the common cold on the Indian Subcontinent.

- Chole - This is a very popular dish made from chickpeas. It is combined with various herbs and spices like cumin, coriander, red pepper, and bay leaves. Different regions of the country have different styles of cooking. Also, some people like to add various vegetables like tomatoes and onions. The chole or chickpeas are usually prepared ahead of time in a slow cooker, or for a faster approach, pressure cooker.

- Rajma - A very popular Indian dish indeed. This is made with kidney beans combined with various spices to give it its taste, color, and texture. This is truly a hearty dish to indulge in. This is one of the most popular beans around.

- Various Dals - Dals are basically lentil-based dishes. There are many types of lentils that can be used and various different spices as well. For example, Chana dal is split chickpeas. These various lentils and spices can combine to make an abundance of different lentil soups that are fully capable of fighting inflammation.

Here are some that can be found in most Indian stores and even international sections of many grocery stores: Udad dal, channa dal, masoor dal, moong dal. These are just a few. All of them are healthy options for an anti-inflammatory diet.

Are you hungry? Well, let's keep going.

- Curry - Curry seems to be one of the most well-known Indian dishes. Curry powder is a combination of various spices, including, coriander, cumin, and turmeric. It often comes in a premixed pouch, but you can certainly make your own. We have mentioned turmeric before because it is a spice that is very popular and effective in fighting chronic inflammation. Some healers have even used it on open wounds for quicker healing.

- Aloo-Mater - This dish is pretty much what is reads, Aloo=Potatos, Mater=Peas. This combination of potatoes, peas, and various spices is a strong antioxidant with anti-inflammatory properties.

- Goby-aloo - Another popular dish. This is a combination of Goby, which is cauliflower and aloo, which are potatoes. Also, mixed with various spices.

- Bhindi - This is one of the most popular dishes in India. It is loved by many for its taste, heralded at the same time for its extreme health benefits. It is a vegetable that is popular in many parts of the world. It is simply known as okra. Okra has a high number of antioxidants and has been known to have anti-inflammatory effects also. The uniqueness of Indian okra is how it is cooked. It is cut up and stir-fried with cumin powder, coriander powder, turmeric, red chili, and mango powder. The result is a tasty treat that is also very healthy. People can add salt as they please, but it must be limited for health reason. In addition to the okra itself, the combination of various spices adds to the health benefits.

- Chaat - Cooked potato patty with peas (called aloo tikkis), on the side, there is yogurt, chickpeas, the sauce made from cilantro, a sauce made from tamarind, and various spices added on. A delicious food often served as popular street food on street side carts called davas.

- Samosas - These particular dishes are fried, so you just have to be careful about how you fry them. They can also be baked in some cases. An outer, tortilla-like covering is shaped in a triangular fashion and filled with potatoes, peas, and various spices like cumin, coriander, and red pepper. Often eaten with a sauce made from tamarind.

- Roti - This is a very common tortilla in India. It is made from whole wheat flour and served with almost any meal.

In this portion, we will talk about some common Indian dishes known as raitas. This is a combination of milk, plain yogurt, and some spices. There are some different kinds of raitas and we will discuss those here.

- Cucumber Raita - This is the base mixture of the milk and plain yogurt. Added in are spices like cumin and coriander. To top it off, we add grated cucumber and voila. We have a delicious and nutritious dish.

- Boondi Raita - This is made in a similar fashion as the cucumber raita. However, instead of cucumber, we added boondi, which is basically fried and puffed chickpea balls.

See a pattern here? A lot of Indian foods are filled with various herbs and spices which are delicious and healthy all at the same time. Most of these meals are not eaten alone. They are usually eaten with rice, preferably brown rice if you're sticking on the diet or various types of tortillas. The most common types in India are called roti, paratha, and naan. The best option of the three is definitely roti. Most Indian food has high fiber and high protein content. You may not even miss meat while you're indulging in some of these culinary delights. Most of the essential herbs and spices that are included in the anti-inflammatory diet are also part of the Indian food diet. There is some confusion now. Is the Mediterranean diet or the Indian diet more anti-inflammatory friendly? They both seem pretty neck and neck as far as the ingredients go. This may just become an argument for the ages. Maybe we can have a blind study done someday. Whatever route you go, you will have a tasty, healthy meal.

Before we go to the next region, we just want to mention Indian Chai. Indian chai is brewed with strong leaves and the addition of ginger, cardamom, cloves, and various other spices based on preference make it a strong anti-inflammatory drink. Indian chai is drunk commonly with many meals, including breakfast and dinner. It is to India what coffee is to the rest of the worlds.

Mexican/Hispanic Food/Latin:

Since Latin America covers so many regions, we will discuss them in one section. Even though food is unique in a lot of areas. We will try to specify if a particular food is found in only a specific area. Take this into account though, a lot of restaurants will add a lot of unnecessary salt and fat to certain dishes. Going to a local fast-food Mexican place may not be the best option. These foods are good, assuming fresh and wholesome ingredients are being used.

- Guacamole and Veggies - Guacamole is made from avocados, which are packed with antioxidants and anti-inflammatory agents. Watch out for those salty chips that you may want to eat with it.

- Vegetarian Burrito - When getting a vegetarian burrito, just make sure to ask for the right ingredients. Ask for black beans and not refried beans. Choose brown rice over white rice. Ask for the salsa and not the sour cream. Finally, ask for some extra vegetables with your burrito. Doing all this will give you a healthy veggie burrito to help combat inflammatory disease.

- Soft tortilla tacos with black beans, lettuce, and tomatoes. Another great option to indulge in.

- Vegetarian Tortilla Soup - Tomato, garlic, and onion broth mixed that submerged with some delicious tortillas. You can also add some black beans. Most people eat this with chicken, but we are leaving that out in order to stick to a vegetarian diet. Sorry, don't get mad at us.

- Red or black bean rice is also a healthy option. Make sure to stay away from refried beans.

- Here is a fun one. How about brown rice with black beans and guacamole.

- Chilled Red Bell Pepper and Habanero Soup - A combination of various spice, garlic, tomatoes, habanero, sweet onion, bell peppers, and olive oil. Once again, a combination of so many foods that fight inflammation.

- This is something we want to mention here because it is very localized to a region. We have spoken extensively about nuts and their anti-inflammatory properties. There are many different types of nuts that fit in these parameters. One thing we have not mentioned yet are Brazil nuts. Since they are very local to Brazil, Bolivia, and Peru, we will mention them here. Brazil nuts have many health benefits, including reducing inflammation. These nuts are very energy-dense and nutritious. Too bad they are not everywhere. That would probably kill their uniqueness though.

- One more thing we will mention here is a fruit called lucuma. It is a Latino superfood. It looks like an avocado from the outside and has the texture of a sweet potato, and has a sweet caramel-like taste. It originated in Peru. We are mentioning here due to its origin and just wanted to make you aware of it. This fruit is filled with antioxidants and has many health benefits, possibly even anti-inflammatory effects.

We just want to prelude the following with an explanation. The next few dishes we are about to describe are popular and even originated in Spain. Based on its Geography, Spain is part of the Mediterranean, so it may be more fitting to have it in that section. The food is also more familiar to that region. However, Spain is also a Spanish speaking country, so we have included it here in this section. Spain also has several distinct dishes. We may be splitting some hairs here, but just wanted to provide an explanation and the method to our madness. That being said, here are some popular Spanish dishes.

- Gazpacho - This is most commonly found in Spain and has many different variations. It is a tomato soup that is served cold, mixed with onions, garlic, olive oil, and a number of local vegetables and spices. This is a popular treat on a hot summer day.
- Pisto Manchego - This is Spanish ratatouille which originates from La Mancha. It is a stew that is made from eggplants, tomatoes, onions, squash, and red peppers. Add some whole wheat bread and you've got a full meal for dinner time.
- Chickpea Salad - A very popular salad in Spain. Chickpeas are great for fighting anti-inflammatory disease and also a great source of protein for vegetarians.
- Spanish Rice - Tomatoes, olive oil, minced garlic, brown rice, with spices like chili powder, turmeric, and cumin. A very popular and healthy dish from the region.
- Spinach and Chickpeas - This dish is very popular in southern Spain. The spinach and chickpeas are accentuated by cumin, paprika, and garlic.
- Marinated Carrots - There is a Spanish word for these, but we can just call them marinated carrots. These are not your average carrots. They are marinated in garlic, oregano, apple cider vinegar, and various other spices. Also, very popular in Southern Spain. Truly, and anti-inflammatory diet lover's dream.
- Smoked Almond Romesco - A combination of tomatoes, peppers, almonds, bread, oil, vinegar, garlic, paprika, and honey.

Asian Food:

Here, we will talk about Asian food. Typically, we think of the greasy chow mein noodles and wonder how that can be healthy. Well, a lot of the food local to the region is not like this. Travel around and see for yourself. For this section, we will include all Asian countries as each separate one would create a lot of sections. Considering this eBook, we have altered some of the recipes too to make them more anti-inflammatory diet-friendly.

- Panang Curry with Vegetables - This is a rich, creamy, spicy, peanut coconut sauce mixed with various vegetables. You can get creative with the vegetables. Some options include red bell peppers and carrots. You can also add tofu for some extra protein. This is a popular Thai curry.
- Our next dish is roasted brussels sprouts and crispy bakes tofu with honey sesame glaze. This is a mouthful. Probably not something you're going to find on a take-out menu either. The brussels sprouts are roasted and put over brown rice with baked tofu added. The top is drizzled with a honey-sesame glaze.
- Spicy Kale and coconut fried rice - Great recipe with a lot of healthy Asian flavors.
- Vegetarian Lettuce Wrap - If you have gone to an Asian restaurant, you may have seen or had these. They are a pretty popular appetizer and maybe even a meal. This is a lettuce leaf topped with sesame-soy soba noodles and quick-pickled veggies. You can also add some edamame hummus. A great addition to any meal.
- Crunchy Thai Peanut Quinoa Salad - This is a combination of quinoa, carrots, cabbage, green onions, snow peas, and cilantro. This is all tossed together in a tasty peanut sauce. Quinoa is also a good source of protein.
- Peanut Slaw with Soba Noodles - This is a colorful slaw with soba noodles and tossed in sesame-ginger peanut sauce. Soba noodles are made from buckwheat. We'll talk some more about Soba noodle recipes.
- Soba Noodles with Miso-Roasted Tomatoes - The cherry tomatoes are roasted in miso, ginger, sesame, lime juice, and honey. All mixed together with the soba noodles.
- Soba with Miso-Glazed Eggplant - Japanese eggplant is good to use with this dish as it is a little sweeter. Mixed with green beans, sesame oil, miso paste, garlic, fresh ginger, spinach, and sliced green onions. All mixed together with the Soba noodles. Everything in this dish is a strong addition to the anti-inflammatory diet.
- Sesame Soba Noodles - Soba Noodles cooked with similar ingredients as before, but with the addition of a hard-boiled egg.
- Are you a fan of sushi? You can still have it. Just substitute white rice for brown rice. Try a salmon and avocado roll.
- Try some veggie sushi options, too. They are plentiful.
- Miso soup, common in most Japanese restaurants. Great option as an anti-inflammatory food.

Italian:

Now things are going to start getting fun. Remember all of those pizza parties you had growing up. Remember that giant lasagna your grandmother made for you. Remember all of those greasy and thick breadsticks. Remember that oily garlic bread. All of that was healthy for you. I mean, it is Italian food and real Italian food is light and healthy and very nutritious. So, go down to the pizza place and order that four-cheese pizza. Order that fully loaded meat pizza with all of the fixes in. And while you are at it, order that extra-large garlic bread with extra marinara sauce. It is healthy for you after all. Of course, none of what we said here is true at all.

It is healthy if it is an authentic Italian food and is made in that region. It actually follows the Mediterranean diet model, which is heralded as one of the healthiest diets in the world. Italian people know how to eat. They use fresh and flavorful ingredients. So, when you go to that pizza place down the road, know that you're not eating authentic, healthy Italian food. The food may be good, but it is anything but healthy. That being said, since authentic Italian does follow that Mediterranean model, it can definitely fit in the lines of an anti-inflammatory diet. People in Italy are some of the healthiest people in the world. Let's talk about some meal and have some tasty Italian food.

- Pasta - Yes, good old-fashioned pasta. Now, we have been heralding against pasta throughout much of this eBook. However, cooking it in the methods used in Italy can create a healthy, fulfilling dish. First of all, cook your pasta al dente, meaning a little firm. This will reduce the glycemic index and reduce carbohydrate absorption. Also, though it is not typically Italian, you can substitute whole grain pasta instead. You can cook this pasta with olive oil, tomatoes, and garlic. This is a tasty pasta dish from the looks of it. And much healthier than the kind you find other places.

- Spaghetti with garlic sauce - Simple spaghetti or whole wheat spaghetti mixed with bits of fresh garlic. You won't be ashamed of having garlic breath when you're in Italy. It is a common staple in this part of the world. It also has a lot of health benefits.

- Garlic-Rosemary Mushrooms - Mushrooms are an amazing source of protein. Plus, garlic and rosemary are two wonderful herbs that will fight hard against inflammatory disease. We are getting quite far here in our Italian dishes. Let's keep going, shall we?

- Hasselback Tomato Caprese Salad - Whole tomatoes, cut, layered in fresh Mozzarella cheese, basil, and a drizzle of balsamic. This is a very tasty appetizer.

- Eggplant Parmesan - This dish is baked and not fried. Rich eggplant provides some essential protein.

- Lemon Herb Salmon with Caponata and Farro - This is a fresh salmon piece, delicious in every way. Topped with herbs and served with brown rice and various vegetables.

- Spaghetti with Broccoli Pesto - A great vegetarian pasta recipe. Spaghetti al dente or whole-grain spaghetti mixed with broccoli, pesto sauce, basil, and Parmigiano-Reggiano. The last one is a hard, granular cheese, which you can leave out if you'd like.

- Whole wheat pizza - It's important to use a base or crust with whole wheat or whole grain. Most crusts made in Italy are thin, so they are not as heavy. Top this lightly with fresh mozzarella cheese, fresh tomatoes, and basil. Delicious pizza that is also very light.

There may now be a three-way tie for healthiest food options with the Mediterranean, Indian, and Italian food. What if you are able to have Mediterranean food for breakfast, Indian food for lunch, and Italian food for dinner? Sounds like a great day to me. We hope that we were able to introduce you to come delicious and healthy Italian dishes. See, Italian food does not have to be fattening and rich with refined carbohydrates. If you use fresh ingredients that are light and healthy, you will get a nutritious meal that you will love. Food is definitely an important staple in Italian culture, and we are very glad to have introduced you to so many healthy meals from that region. We hope this will satisfy your taste buds. Remember also to get creative. Think about the various ingredients that you may have used over the years that are common in Italy. Some of these include oregano, parsley, basil, olive oil, and garlic. Think of your own creative recipes and meal plans that will satisfy the anti-inflammatory diet. We have spoken in-depth about the various food groups involved in the specific diet. Use this information to help you create your own works of art. Good luck with creating delicious meal plans that are also healthy. I think there are enough meal plans in this book alone to last you a whole year. It is amazing how many dishes can be made from all of the various foods and we are just barely scratching the surface.

We are glad you were able to take this little trip around the world with us. Thank you so much for doing so. We had a blast discussing various meals from around the globe that will fit into the anti-inflammatory diet. We got a little hungry writing this chapter. It was amazing learning about all of these amazing foods that exist in the world. The writers of a book often learn just as much as the readers. As you can see, the anti-inflammatory diet is a worldwide phenomenon, whether the world realizes it or not. Even if certain recipes do not go by the name of the anti-inflammatory diet, the food choices they use certainly do.

Once again, if you are a heavy meat-eater, you may have been disappointed in this chapter a little bit. There is certainly a lot of great food in the world that includes meat. We would love for you to learn about them. However, for this book, we are still sticking to vegan and vegetarian foods. No matter how tempting some meal plans may look. There may be a lot of cross-over from one region to another, especially if those regions are in close proximity. Our hope is that, in this chapter, we were able to cover most of the major areas in the world and give you a good understanding of the anti-inflammatory diet as it relates to culinary treats from around the globe. Thank you again for joining us on this journey.

Chapter 7: Setting Up A Schedule: Taking Action

Now we have the knowledge, time to put in the work. We have discussed the anti-Inflammatory diet in great detail. But, here's the deal, none of this information provided will mean anything if you do nothing with it. Period! Knowledge with action is ultimately meaningless. We don't say that to be mean, just to be truthful. If you are ready to move forward with the diet plan, then let's take action and start incorporating it into your life. The best way to do so is by making your own personal schedule. With this schedule, we will create lists of specific foods and meals you can eat to satisfy the diet. Of course, nothing has to be set in stone. This can simply be a guideline.

Let's get started by producing a weeklong schedule to give us an idea of how it can work. We will base this on a regular Sunday to Saturday schedule. Let's bring all of this full-circle and start incorporating it into your life. This is just a sample schedule. Obviously, you will make your own as you see fit. It is your schedule after all. Once again, this is just a guideline. Use it as inspiration, but you don't have to follow it to a T. We will move along with the assumption that you are just starting the anti-inflammatory diet. How about we call this a story? A week in the life of you.

Sunday:

The start of the week for most people. This is the day that sets up the rest of the week and how it will go. You commonly hear people say that Sunday should set the tone for the rest of the six days. This is very true and the diet you create will set up your cravings for the week to come. Start your Sunday off with some hearty meals. Start your week off the right way and kick off your anti-inflammatory diet in high fashion. What happened up to this point is history. Today, we start something new. Let's begin, shall we?

- Start off your morning with a good breakfast. First things first, you probably have not drunken anything all night. Start off your day by getting hydrated. Drink a nice tall glass of lemon water. You can also add some apple cider vinegar if you please. A cup of green tea is a great thing to have for some energy and nutrients. A piece of fruit like a banana or apple and then a bowl of oatmeal with raw honey and some blueberries. Add some raisins to the top of that. A light, but hearty breakfast.

- For a mid-morning snack, indulge in some blueberries and almonds. A filling snack that will provide protein and antioxidants. Remember also to keep hydrated with some water. Always keep some water with you. It is an important addition to any anti-inflammatory diet.

- For lunch, have a walnut salad with cranberries and some vinaigrette dressing. In the afternoon is where tiredness usually kicks in. People will often make this worse by eating a greasy meal at lunch. Lethargy will really start setting in at this point and there is still so much of the day left. Instead, have a meal that's filling and energizing all at the same time. A walnut salad will definitely fill you up, but not weigh you down. Compliment this with a glass of freshly squeezed orange juice. A piece of fruit like an apple can also be included.

- For a late afternoon snack, enjoy something like a banana or other favorite fruit. A late afternoon snack is important in order to keep up your energy levels and keep up your metabolism. Drink another glass of water while you are at it. This will keep you going until dinner time.

- For dinner, eat at least a couple of hours before bed. Perhaps a nice grilled salmon with some vegetables are a good option. Some carrots, celery, and potatoes will make it a filling and healthy meal. You will end your day feeling satiated, but not bloated. The main goal is to not feel awful after eating it. Plus, you definitely do not want to feel overly full right before bedtime.

- You may still be a little active after dinner, depending on your schedule. It is good to eat a light snack prior to bedtime. Maybe a nice cup of Greek yogurt will do you good. Having a light, healthy snack before bedtime will keep you from getting hungry overnight. It will also keep your blood sugars from fluctuating too much.

Sunday was a good day for our diets and our palates. We really stuck to the anti-inflammatory diet in this case. This was a great initial first step. It is just the first day and we have a long way to go. Remember though our week is just kicking off, so let's keep moving and let's stay focused.

Monday:

If you are like most people, Monday is the start of the workweek for you. Of course, there are several non-regular schedules that are becoming more and more common. For this schedule, we will assume you have a 9-5, Monday-Friday workweek. Our busy schedules during the week filled with work, family, hobbies, and more can make it seem impossible to stick to a routine diet. It can be done though. It is time to get our Monday started and begin tackling the workweek.

- Rise up early for your day so you have time to make yourself a good breakfast before work. It is also advised that you prepare what you can the night before to save you some time in the morning. For this morning, we will have a bowl of fruit, walnuts, Egg whites with some turmeric, and a glass of fresh apple juice. Start your workday off with some fresh food and be ready to attack whatever comes your way. Not attack in the literal sense. Of course, before you eat this, get hydrated with a nice glass of lemon water. Still have that caffeine craving, make yourself another cup of green tea. Regular coffee works too, but green tea is usually a healthier option.

- You are having a busy Monday morning coming back from the weekend. You are feeling more energized than you usually do. The first couple of hours go by quickly. For a mid-morning snack, get a nice blueberry smoothie from the juice place in the lobby of your work. If you have one of course. If not, improvise with something else. Just have something light and refreshing. Avoid that vending machine though. It's evil.

- The afternoon rush is hitting at work. People are coming to you for all sorts of things that need to get done. Another couple of hours passes by without a breeze. For lunch, we can go Mediterranean. How about a large Greek salad? Greek salads usually come with a lot of fix-ins. It will be a satisfying lunch and you really won't need anything else except maybe a glass of water. If you're craving a sweeter drink, consider some type of yogurt drink. Keep it Mediterranean for now.

- The workday is going along well after your healthy lunch. You still feel energized and ready to go. However, it is late afternoon again and you are probably hungry once more. It is time for the afternoon snack and luckily, you have something on you. It is a banana. After eating it, you are ready to finish out your day. Your Monday at work ends well. You were busy, but you stuck to your diet plan. Good for you.

- When you arrive home, it is time for dinner. What will you have though? There are so many options. Let's stick to the Mediterranean diet. It has been the theme for today. How about some hummus with pita bread, a bulgur salad, and some type of fresh juice? Perhaps, pineapple juice will complement everything. This is a delicious meal and you feel great afterward. Time to relax and get some things prepared for tomorrow.

- For a late-night snack, let's grab a handful of walnuts. Those are always quite delicious and filled with Omega-3 fatty acids, which are needed to fight inflammation. Shortly after this, it is time for bed. Congratulations! That is day number two down and we are on a roll!

Our Monday has been successful. We had a full workday, but we stuck to our diet and were able to eat multiple types of food. Our week is going pretty well so far. We can lay in bed at night knowing that we ate well, we feel good, and don't have excessing heartburn. Like we did so many times in the past. Feel proud of yourself. You deserve it.

Tuesday:

We are onto the third day of our week and we are feeling pretty good. So far, it has been easy sticking to our diet plan. We sleep really well at night. We feel good during the day. We are waking up in less pain and discomfort and we have accomplished so much already. It has been a blast.

- Now, for breakfast, let's change things up a little bit. We will still start off our day with a nice tall glass of lemon water. We will drink a green smoothie, which is very filling. Plus, we will eat a banana. Let's also have something different from green tea. How about a nice cup of turmeric tea? We will try that this morning. Once again, you are feeling energized. You are ready to take on another workday. You arrive at work and all of your friends notice a kick in your step. You're boss notices this, too.

- After completing all of your morning tasks, you are feeling hungry for a snack. Luckily, you have a container of strawberries in your lunch bag, so you indulge in some of those. The freshness of those strawberries gives you another kick in your step. You continue to feel good. The morning continues to pass by quickly and you remain busy and focused.

- For lunch, you kind of feel like going out. You want to stick to your diet plan though. Never worry though because down the street is an excellent gourmet sandwich shop. When you arrive there, you notice that they have a veggie sandwich that uses a black bean patty. This is interesting, so let's get that. With the sandwich, we can add some lettuce, tomatoes, red onions, vinegar, red pepper, black pepper, and olives. We will leave out the salt, but the sandwich still tastes pretty good. It has been easy to stay on track with the food so far. This lunch was exceptional. Of course, let's wash it down with some water. Afterward, you go back to work.

- You get back to work after lunch and after a couple of hours, you get hungry again. You look in your bag to see what you have available and find some cut up oranges. A good healthy snack to help you finish out the workday. The rest of the afternoon goes off well. You did have some fires to put out, but because of the extra energy you have been having, it is easy for you to do so.

- After you go home, you are ready to have some dinner. You get a call, though. It is a friend asking you to come to a party he is having. You have not seen this friend in weeks, so you really want to see him. But you don't want to mess up your diet. You decide to go, though. It's important to see your friend. When you get there, there is nothing really for you to eat that satisfies the anti-inflammatory diet. It is not your friend's fault though because he doesn't know about your diet. You decide to suck it up and see what they have. Mostly, it is greasy food like chicken wings and pizza. There is a small veggie tray you can eat from, so that's something. You take a few bites, but it certainly does not fill you up. You look around for more food, but there is nothing else you see. You will still be at the party for another hour at least, so you really want to eat. You also don't want to seem rude to your friend. Well, there is no other choice at this point. You are at a party and want to enjoy time with your friend. I guess we can cheat on the diet a little bit. Have a slice of pizza and some chicken wings. The last few days have been good so celebrate a little bit. Instead of soda though, you just have plain water. You don't want to drink that sugary drink that will provide no nutritional value. You have a fun time for the rest of the party.

- When you get home, it's still a couple of hours until you go to bed. You decide a good snack to have are some carrot sticks. There taste pretty good with a little bit of lime squirted on them. You also decide to drink some lemon water with a touch of apple cider vinegar. This has always done wonders for your acid reflux, which just might occur because of the pizza. You had a couple of more slices than you wanted to. It's ok though. Tomorrow is another day.

You end the night feeling a little bad, but overall, it was a good day. Plus, you got to see your friend and spend some time with them. It is important to maintain a good lifestyle while eating well, too. We are a total of three days into the week and things are going pretty well. It's time to call it a night and get ready for the next day. Good job getting through another day. Let's keep moving.

Wednesday:

You wake up on Wednesday morning and are feeling pretty good. A little bit tired because you did not sleep as well because of the greasy food you ate at night. It's ok though to indulge occasionally. Today is a new day. We shall see how it goes.

- At the start of the morning, you are feeling extra thirsty, so you make a taller glass of lemon water. It tastes pretty refreshing for the most part. For breakfast, you have another bowl of oatmeal topped with raisins, blueberries, raw honey, and bananas. Also, you go back to drinking your green tea. The turmeric tea did not taste as good. It is okay though because not everything will satisfy your palate. You also have a cup of fresh yogurt with strawberries. A healthy and filling breakfast to start your Wednesday. It's time to make up from yesterday and get this day going right.

- After arriving at work, things are quite busy and hectic. It is okay because you have everything under control. You also have the energy to handle everything thrown at you. It's been so busy that you almost forgot your midmorning snack. Lucky for you though, there are some walnuts in your desk that you can have. They taste quite good and they give you the energy you need until lunchtime. You are able to tackle the rest of the morning with ease. Your boss appreciates your hard work.

- Lunchtime comes around and you made yourself a sandwich with whole wheat bread, lettuce, tomatoes, red onions, and pickles. You are ready to indulge until your coworkers interrupt you. They want you to come to have lunch with them. You really don't want to because you already cheated on your diet the night before. However, you realize they are going to have lunch at an Indian restaurant. It will be pretty easy to stick to your diet there and you remember that this particular place makes their food pretty fresh. You decide to go ahead and eat there. When you arrive, you scope out what they have. All of it looks pretty good, but you stick to the vegetarian portions. You fill up your plate with kidney beans, chickpeas, lentil soup, and potatoes. You also grab some whole wheat tortillas. This will be quite a satisfying meal indeed. For a drink, you just get some water. When you start eating the spicy food, you realize that water may not be sufficient enough to take away the burning sensation in your mouth. They have healthy yogurt drinks on the menu, so you decide to get one. It tastes sour, but pretty good overall with the meal. It was a nice lunch and you feel pretty good afterward. You stuck to your diet and spent time with your coworkers. After this lunch, everyone goes back to work to continue the day.

- When you get back to work, you immediately begin on your tasks that need to be completed for that day. There is much to do but you can handle it. When late afternoon hits, it is time for your snack. Since you have built it into your routine, your body almost knows by itself when this time comes. You are too full still for that sandwich you made, instead, there is a container of raspberries in your bag. You eat these and feel satisfied. You are able to finish out the rest of your day with ease. It is finally time to finally go home and rest.

- When you get home, you wonder about dinner. You had a fairly big lunch and are still pretty full. However, you decide to make some tabbouleh and eat some whole wheat pita bread. This is a light and refreshing meal. It is still pretty early, so you decide to go to the gym. There are some extra calories to burn off today. Indian and Mediterranean food. A pretty good combination to satisfy the anti-inflammatory diet.

- After the gym, you sit and watch some television for a while. Before retiring to bed, you eat a nice light snack. There is still some Greek yogurt leftover. This is your perfect late-night snack, especially when you add some blueberries. After eating this, you go to bed and end your day. There was a wide variety of food that you ate on this day and it all satisfied the anti-inflammatory diet plan.

We are officially past the halfway point of the week and things are going well. In fact, they are going pretty great. A lot of your eating habits are starting to fit into your routine by this point. It is important though to not let temptation get to you. Also, it is important to do your research when determining what food is best for you. It can be tedious and exhausting, but it will be worth it because you will feel much better. You probably have already noticed the difference in your energy levels by sticking with the anti-inflammatory diet. Let's keep going and finish the rest of the week strong. You are doing great so far!

Thursday:

Okay, it is now the fifth day of the week. You get up early once more. You notice that by this day, getting up earlier is much easier than it was before. It is a combination of training your body and also having more energy from good food. Not only does a good diet help you function better during the day, but it also helps you have a more relaxing sleep at night. A proper diet works wonders for your ability to function, as you may have noticed already. It is Thursday already. This week is going by quite fast. Let's see how it goes.

- Once again, you start your day by drinking a fresh glass of lemon water. This drink always satisfies your thirst and gives you some energy first thing in the morning. You decide this morning that you want some extra protein. You make some egg white with tomatoes, green peppers, crushed black pepper, and turmeric. For a side, you eat a bowl of roasted almonds. You also drink a fresh green smoothie. You're not really craving the green tea today. Of course, the green smoothie is quite filling, so you are not able to finish it all at once. No worries though, because you can put it into a to-go cup. After this, you are ready to start your day. You head out your front and start heading to work.

- When you arrive at work, things are extra busy, so you immediately have to jump into action. There are many fires to put out today. Luckily, the extra protein is kicking in to help you keep moving. You are a little late due to the hecticness of the day. However, you still make time for your midmorning snack. You decide to go to the refrigerator and grab that green smoothie you made in the morning. It still tastes pretty good and gives you the strength to keep moving. The last couple of hours before lunch are brutal. You never really get a chance to sit down. Your mind and body are moving constantly. Good thing you had that extra protein in the morning.

- Come lunchtime, you are ready to eat again. Just so it didn't go to waste, you packed the sandwich for yourself that you did not eat the day before. It is still fresh and tastes pretty good. All of the vegetables with the whole wheat bread satisfies your diet plan well. For a beverage, you just wash it down with some water. There is a problem though. You are still quite hungry and that sandwich did not fill you up. There is still some celery in your lunch bag, but you want to save that for later. You know that you are still going to have a busy afternoon, so you want to make sure you are full. Your only option right now is to get something from the vending machine. That evil vending machine. It is filled with nothing but salty snacks and candies. It has been a good week for you, so you decide a bag of chips won't hurt you. They taste pretty good and you definitely notice the extra salt. After lunch is finished, you get back to work promptly. Your body does not notice the unhealthy snack, so you keep moving and get things done. It is quite a busy afternoon, but you are able to handle everything well.

- It is late afternoon once more and you are ready for your late afternoon snack. You finish the celery sticks in your lunch bag, and they get you through the rest of the day. The busy Thursday workday is over. Finally, it is time to go home.

- When you arrive home you get ready for dinner. You want to get a little bit creative. For tonight, you make a burrito with black beans, tomatoes, lettuce, and onions. The first one tastes pretty good, so you make another one. You also decide to make some guacamole. It all tastes pretty good and fills you up. At this time, you have been on the anti-inflammatory diet for about five days and have tried three different ethnic foods. You decide at this point that you will experiment more regularly with different foods to try many new things. Your old diet of hotdogs, burgers, and pizza is a thing of the past. This will also keep you from getting bored with the diet. You decide for dinner to drink some coconut water. First time trying it and it tastes good. You are excited to keep moving and keep getting better. There is nothing stopping you now.

- After working on the computer for a while, you have a late-night snack. You still have some cut up avocado leftover from the guacamole. You decide to eat that. It is good, but also a little bland for you. You add some black peppers, and it helps a little bit. You are able to finish it and get some essential nutrients. The biggest thing you have noticed with your new diet plan is that with the variety of foods available, you do not feel like you are missing anything. Today was quite a good protein day overall.

So far, it has been five full days and you are sticking to your diet well. You don't miss your old way of life and are enjoying the direction you are going with your health. This is very important. Having a purpose and seeing results is a great motivator. We will continue on to Friday and see how we can finish off this week.

Friday:

- It is Friday morning and the weekend will be upon us soon enough. When you wake up in the morning, you have a craving for something sweet. First things first, you drink a glass of lemon water and get hydrated. This will be your staple from now on. A full glass of lemon water every morning. No matter what diet plan you follow, being hydrated is essential. After this, you grab a muffin, which you have been craving since you woke up. Luckily, it is a bran muffin, so not too bad. It still has a lot of sugar in it. In addition, you have a banana and some yogurt with a cup of green tea. Overall, not too bad of a start for your day. After eating, you head to work. It is Friday, so all of the tasks of the day are needing to be completed before the weekend starts. It is a busy morning indeed with nonstop meetings, emails, phone calls, and writing. When you finally get a chance to stop and eat, your boss calls you into his office. He compliments you on your work this past week and offers to give you more responsibility. This is an honor for you and could lead to bigger things in the near future. After the meeting, you quickly get back to work.

- After a few minutes, you remember about your morning snack. You quickly grab some coconut water and some pecans from your bag. They taste pretty good, but you are also pretty close to lunch, so you only have a few. At least with the busy schedule, you were still able to stick to your meal plan. The rest of the morning goes by quickly as you get back to doing the work you need. You really need to complete all of the pending tasks before the weekend starts or your Monday will be impossible to deal with.

- For lunch, you are craving a salad. There is a good place down the road that has pretty good fresh salads. When you arrive there, you order one with green beans, spinach, lettuce, red onions, cucumbers, and parsley. You top it off with an avocado dressing that they have. All of it tastes wonderful. You are happy with lunch. You wash it down with a glass of beets juice that they make fresh there. The lunch was very filling and tasted quite good, too. You feel energized once more after this lunch and ready to get back to work. It is still a little early, so you decide to take a quick walk. The fresh air feels good after you have been stuck in an office all day long.

- The afternoon is filled with more meetings, emails, writing, and putting out many fires before the weekend. It has been a busy Friday and it was only halfway done. After a couple of hours, it is now time for a late afternoon snack. This time, you have a mixture of roasted cashews, almonds, and peanuts. You have learned by now to prepare a few things the night before to have on hand. The snacks fill you up for the rest of the day until you are ready to go home. When your workday ends, your boss calls you into his office. He compliments you on a good week. He states that your work rate has improved tremendously all due to the new diet. Okay, well maybe we're taking things too far here. Whatever the case, your workweek is completed, and you are ready to enjoy your weekend. You get a few final things closed out, say goodbye to a few people, and then you are on your way.

- When you get home, you decide to order out. You go for Mediterranean food again and get a Greek salad, vegetarian pita sandwich with falafel made from chickpeas, and some hummus with pita bread. The pita bread will probably last you through the weekend. All the food tasted exceptional and you still have the energy to do a few things. You decide to meet up with your friend at the movies. It has been a long week and you deserve a good night out. When you get there, you strongly resist their urge to get popcorn or candy. Your friend gorged on some junk food while you continued to resist. Honestly, you aren't even craving it at this point. The movie was nice and now you are ready to go back home. Before this, you and your friend have a chat about your new diet plan. He seems impressed and asks you more questions about it. You explain to him all of the various food groups and meals you can eat. You also explain to him about the increased energy levels and overall feelings of well-being. He seems interested in starting it someday as well. You both agree to follow a similar schedule starting Sunday. This should be a lot of fun.

- After arriving back home, you decide to have some carrots dipped in the hummus you have from before. It is a tasty little snack. After this, you end your night and are ready for another weekend. You fall asleep pretty quickly as it has been quite a busy day.

This has been a really good week for you so far. You have really been doing your part in fighting off inflammatory disease, simply by eating a healthy diet. I hope you are feeling good about yourself so far. You have done an impressive job sticking to your diet, even though you are extremely busy. You have also resisted a lot of temptations. There is just one day left in the week. Time to start day number seven of the anti-inflammatory diet. Good Luck!

Saturday:

The weekend is now upon you and you did a great job sticking to your diet during the week. Even with your busy work schedule, you made the time to always eat healthy meals. On Saturday morning, you sleep in a little bit. The movie ended somewhat late, so you also got to bed later than usual.

- When you wake up, as usual, you start your day with a fresh glass of lemon water. This has become almost a habit for you. You often crave this refreshing drink first thing in the morning now. For good reason, too. It is a great drink to start off your day. After this, you start on your hearty breakfast. Just a week earlier, your Saturday morning breakfast consisted of greasy eggs, bacon, and sausage. This morning, all you are craving are egg whites with spinach, green peppers, and black pepper. Also, on the side, you have some fresh cut up strawberries, blueberries, and a whole banana. To drink, you have a cup of green tea. A far cry from what you used to have. An impressive change and a positive move towards fighting inflammatory disease. You indulge in your Saturday morning breakfast. Even though it is the weekend, you will not shy away from your commitment.

- After breakfast, you go to the gym, grocery shopping, and run a few other errands. About midmorning, you remember to grab a snack. You get a fresh-squeezed orange juice from one of your favorite juice places. Once again, the prior week, you were getting your energy from coffee, sodas, or energy drinks. Now, you are getting it naturally from the foods you eat.

- In the early afternoon, while still running errands, you stop to have lunch at an Indian Restaurant you have fallen in love with. For lunch, you have some whole wheat tortillas, potatoes with peas and various spices, curry, kidney beans, and some rice. They do not have brown rice, so you must settle for white rice. Overall, the meal is very tasty and quite healthy. All of the mixtures of the flavors are very satisfying to your palate. It really makes you not even miss eating meat. At least for the time being. After lunch, you continue with your day. It is a busy Saturday, but you have the energy to handle it just fine.

- Around late afternoon time, you grab a snack, which is a small fresh protein shake you get from a local juice place. It is quite good. You opted for more than a snack because you will still be running errands for a while and need the energy. It still takes a couple more hours of running around in order to finish everything you need to do.

- Finally, you arrive back home and are ready for dinner. While you were out, you picked up a few things for the evening and the rest of the week. For dinner, you decide to make whole wheat pasta and some parsley salad. For a drink, you opt for some regular water. It is a great dinner for you that you really enjoyed. You look at all of the things you bought while you were out and are ready to get the week started and continue your newfound diet plan. The anti-inflammatory diet is definitely serving you well. After dinner, you relax and watch TV for a while. It has been a long day and you are tired.

- Well, it's late at night and its time to go to bed soon. Before that though, you call your friend and set up your schedule for the following week. You will be his support system and he will hopefully be yours, too. You guys are able to plot out your whole week and are optimistic about how it will turn out. The first week went great, so no doubt the second week will be even better. For a late-night snack tonight, why don't you indulge a little bit. You have definitely earned it. How about some avocado ice cream? After that, time to go to bed. The week is completed. Well done!

Well, you made it through the first week on the new anti-inflammatory diet plan and you did great. Except for a few detours here and there, you stuck to your diet very well. Obviously, this was an exaggerated meal plan and just used as a guideline. We hope that it at least provides a good illustration of how it can fit into your schedule. We realize that your schedule is your own and you will have to incorporate the diet in your own way based on your available times and your own taste buds. Our hope is that we have encouraged you to set up your own schedule and include this new plan into your life, especially if you are already suffering from chronic inflammation or inflammatory disease. Once again, this is not a one-size-fits-all plan. We also advise you to seek out a professional when making life-altering changes, especially those that affect your body processes.

As was portrayed by this story, one can truly improve their overall health and livelihood by changing something as simple as the food they ingest. We hope that your own story has a similar result to the one we told. Bottom line is this: You have to take action in order to start making improvements. Having knowledge does not mean anything unless you are ready to use it. Good luck and thank you for helping us bring all of this full circle.

Chapter 8: The Popular Diet

So far in this book, we have talked about Inflammatory disease, how dangerous it can be, and how to prevent and even resolve it with some lifestyle changes like the anti-inflammatory diet. We went in-depth on the diet and included many different foods, both locally and from around the world that follows the anti-inflammatory diet. We still encourage you to get creative with your own meal plans as well. Cooking is an art form, so have fun with it.

We also helped you set up a schedule. Well, sort of. We made an example of a schedule for someone who may be changing over to an anti-inflammatory diet. You can follow that one or change it as you wish based on your own schedule and palate. We just hope that we helped illustrate how the diet can fit into your lives and how it can replace certain unhealthy foods you may have been eating. We really enjoyed giving you all of this useful information and we sincerely hope that is able to help you get on the right track as far as healthy eating. Diet is crucial in fighting many chronic illnesses, and the anti-inflammatory diet has been found to reduce chronic inflammation, or inflammatory disease, which leads to a lot of chronic illnesses. We hope that you will not only read this book once but use it as a reference over and over again. The information can be referenced on a regular basis.

As you can see, the concepts of the anti-inflammatory diet are quite simple. You eat the right foods and you will get the right results. What is important is that it takes effort, patience, persistence, determination, and sacrifice. You have it in you, now make it happen.

Before we close out this Book, we want to share some stories about how the anti-inflammatory diet has helped so many people throughout history and modern times. We will also share stories of people who have lived a vegetarian or vegan dietary lifestyle. We mentioned before how you should not follow something just because a bunch of famous people is doing it. We still believe this one hundred percent. However, we feel that by showing examples of well-known people eating a proper anti-inflammatory diet can truly help shine a light on it. To be fair, many of these people were following an anti-inflammatory diet and may not have even realized it. Maybe you have followed it to a certain degree also. If so, we encourage you to continue. The reason we used famous and more well-known people as an example is that it has more of an impact. A neighbor down the street who prevented himself from getting a heart attack may not be as useful or appealing to the masses. We do applaud that person though if this is the case for them. Let's get started.

Mike Tyson:

Well-known heavyweight boxer and media personality Mike Tyson was once the most famous athlete in the country. Maybe even the most famous person in the world period. He captivated the world with his speed strength and style. The youngest heavyweight champion of all time. During his time as a boxer, he certainly was no vegetarian and was not following the anti-inflammatory diet. During his reign, not much was known about the protein available in non-meat foods. At this time though, Tyson was working out constantly and could probably eat whatever he wanted. Tyson admitted that he was not sure if he could have sustained a vegan lifestyle while boxing, but he says it might have been a possibility as many gladiators of the past were vegans or vegetarians.

After he stopped fighting and was not training either, Mike Tyson's weight ballooned up. At one point, he was weighing over 300 pounds. Eventually, he would change to a more plant-based diet and this would lead him to lose over 100 pounds and get back down to his healthy weight. Mike is a great example of how the vegan/vegetarian, and in turn, anti-inflammatory diet can have a positive impact on someone's life. Mike Tyson is still able to work out hard when he wants to. We applaud him for his accomplishments.

Kevin Smith:

Well-known comedian and film producer who has worked on many projects. He is famously known for the Jay and Silent Bob movies. Smith has had issues with his health off and on for decades, especially in relation to his weight which has gone up and down constantly. At one time, he weighed over 400 pounds.

In 2018, Kevin Smith suffered a major heart attack after performing a stand-up comedy show. Luckily for Mr. Smith, he was rushed to the hospital and had emergency surgery, which saved his life. He had total blockage of one of his arteries, which would have been fatal if not treated.

After this frightening incident, Kevin Smith, with the guidance of his doctor, went on a plant-based diet starting with potatoes and then slowly incorporating other foods week by week. This new diet plan served Smith well as he has lost well over 50 pounds and is a whole new person. He continues to maintain his healthy vegan diet until this day. Kevin Smith's story is a perfect example of how things were taken way too far with the ignoring of his health problems. His story also perfectly illustrates how the combination of modern medicine and lifestyle changes can work together to save someone's life. Obviously, Kevin Smith needed extreme measures to save his life once he had a heart attack. However, afterward, he has worked hard on his diet to assure it won't happen again. We congratulate Mr. Kevin Smith for his great work on and off-screen.

Penn Jillette:

Penn Jillette is a famous magician, illusionist, and media personality. He appears on various news channels on a regular basis. He is part of the popular duo of Penn and Teller. Penn Jillette has a great act, or several great acts, that he does. He can make almost anything disappear, even parts of himself.

He did just that a few years back. Back in 2015, Penn Jillette ended up in the Emergency Room with extremely high blood pressure. He was also found to have 90% blockage in one of his arteries. He was a ticking time bomb for sure. He wanted to make a major change in his life for himself and his family. He knew that he could not be there for his kids and maintain the dietary habits that he had.

With the help of his doctor, Mr. Jillette went on an extreme diet. He ate nothing but potatoes with no salt or other additives. Just plain potatoes and that's all. After two weeks, he was already down several pounds. He slowly began incorporating other stews and vegetables into his diet in order to receive other nutrients. This was similar to the diet plan that Kevin Smith had. In fact, Penn Jillette was the inspiration for Kevin Smith. After a few months, Mr. Jillette was down over a hundred pounds. It was an amazing transformation, to say the least. Mr. Jillette continues to maintain his weight and lives his busy lifestyle.

If the anti-inflammatory diet is good enough for them, it is certainly good enough for all of us. Just so we are clear, all of the people we have described so far lost a significant amount of weight by changing their diet plans. This has worked out great for them, but they also had help. We want to make it clear that losing drastic amounts of weight quickly can be extremely dangerous if not monitored closely. For this reason, we always advise seeking the help of a professional when doing so. It will give you peace of mind also. The diet plans that the above people followed also follow the anti-inflammatory diet.

Let's talk now about some famous athletes. These high caliber performers earned their accolades while also maintaining a healthy vegan/vegetarian diet. We will share some examples below.

Hannah Teter:

Hannah Teter is an American snowboarder. She won the gold medal in the 2006 Winter Olympic Games and multiple other championships throughout the years. She has been following a plant-based diet for some time now and she states it has made her feel better than ever. It has opened her mind to so many new things as an athlete. Hannah Teter has always appreciated protecting the environment, which led her to a vegan, plant-based diet. Since turning to a plant-based diet, she states that she feels stronger physically, mentally, and emotionally. Hannah continues to compete as a professional snowboarder.

David Haye:

We spoke about professional boxer Mike Tyson. Now, we will discuss a more recent champion in David Haye. David Haye was a very successful cruiserweight, winning multiple titles. After he researched the effects of a vegan diet on the healing process after suffering a serious shoulder injury, he realized that he did not need to eat meat to have the strength he needed to compete. He states that he has a full-time chef and nutritionist who help make sure he gets all of his nutrients while following a plant-based diet. David Haye competed until 2018, then retired from the ring. If professional athletes can benefit from an anti-inflammatory style diet, then so can the rest of us.

Barney Du Plessis:

Who the heck is this? Well, if you are a bodybuilding fan, you probably know who it is. He is the world's first vegan bodybuilder and was Mr. Universe in 2014. Du Plessis went vegan in 2013 after having a growing list of health concerns. He also retired from bodybuilding after this. When he changed his diet, it changed his fitness in a radical way. He feels that with a vegan diet, it allows him to train half as much, but still get better results. He feels that he gets more GMO-free and organic food by avoiding meat. After turning Vegan in 2013 and almost ending his career in 2013, he went on to win the prestigious Mr. Universe in 2014. That is a great story if we've ever heard one. Du Plessis and his partner are now doing their part to spread the positive message of a vegan diet. The way to a happy, healthy, and prosperous life.

Nate Diaz:

Nate Diaz is a mixed martial artist who competes for the largest promotion for the sport in the world. He adopted a vegan lifestyle when he was 18. He was inspired by his older brother, who was already competing. He says that the vegan diet has made him a stronger and better fighter, plus it also makes him feel better the day after.

Meagan Duhamel:

Meagan Duhamel is an Olympic medalist pair skater and a four-time world champion. Meagan switched to eating whole grains, fruits, and vegetables when she read about a vegan diet in a book she found in 2008. She read it cover to cover and was amazed by what she read. She stopped eating animal products after that and continued to compete at the highest level.

Gama Pehalvan:

We are really going into the annals of history for this particular person. Gama Pehalvan was born Ghulam Mohammad Baksh. Pehalvan was a world-class wrestler from India during the late 1800s and early 1900s who is often considered one of the greatest wrestlers in the history of time. He inspired many people down the line, including Bruce Lee.

On a regular day, Gama Pehalvan would wrestle about forty of his fellow wrestlers, perform five thousand squats and three thousand pushups. This was his daily training session. One of the most unique things about Pehalvan was his diet. While it was not solidly a vegan or vegetarian diet, it mostly was and also followed anti-inflammatory diet of today. Here's a brief look at his diet. It would consist of 10 liters of milk, mixed with crushed almond paste. Three buckets of seasonal fruits and various fruit juices. He did eat chicken, so we can't say that he had a vegetarian diet. Of course, some people still call chicken part of the vegetarian diet. A milder form of it. That is for other people to decide, not us. Nevertheless, his diet and lifestyle truly illustrate how fruits, vegetables, and dairy products promote health and energy.

Venus Williams:

Venus Williams is a famous tennis player. She is arguably the greatest female tennis player of all time. After some health issues in 2011 related to an auto-immune disease, Venus Williams decided to adopt a vegan diet based on the advice from her doctors. This would continue her performance on the court, which is what she wanted. After trying it, she fell in love and has stuck to it ever since. Venus Williams continues to dominate on the court to this day. A great example of an anti-inflammatory/vegan diet helping someone with an auto-immune disorder. This has really been the basis for our eBook today. Congratulations to Venus Williams for sticking to her diet plan.

Scott Jurek:

Scott Jurek is an ultramarathon runner and holds many personal records. While Jurek was in college, he saw multiple people suffering from health defects while he was attending physical therapy school. His mother also had multiple sclerosis. He saw veganism as a solution to many of the chronic diseases that were in his family's history. This was a long-term decision made by Jurek. One that he is very proud of. Being vegan still allows Jurek to perform at very high levels.

Jermain Defoe:

Jermain Defoe is a footballer/soccer player and one of the best goal scorers in the league. He believes that switching over to a vegan diet helped him in a big way during his comeback in the sport.

These are some amazing stories of some of the top-level athletes in the world and how they followed and even promoted a largely anti-inflammatory and vegan/vegetarian diet. If it allowed them to still compete at the highest level, there must be something great about it.
Since we discussed some high-level athletes, let's also discuss some celebrities who often have to be in top form in order to do what they are best at.

Ellen DeGeneres:

Ellen is truly someone who is popular with the masses. She seems to be everywhere. In order to do this, she has to take good care of herself. She has to be in top form all of the time. She does it not so much for health reasons, but for animal rights. However, the proof is in the pudding and Ellen continues to live a high-level lifestyle on the vegan diet.

Usher:

Usher's father died of a heart attack in 2008. This inspired Usher to change his dietary habits to veganism. He wanted to adopt a healthier lifestyle and not have the same fate as his father.

These are just a couple of celebrities who have adopted a vegan lifestyle for various reasons. More often than not, it is due to a health concern, either imminent or probable. There is no denying that a vegan diet has so many health benefits considering there is example after example of it helping somebody. There are even real-life examples of the anti-inflammatory diet helping someone with chronic inflammation. Take Venus Williams as an example. According to her, she was able to get past her auto-immune disorder by changing her diet. A great story, indeed. There is also growing evidence that foods which fight inflammation work well to negate inflammatory disease and other chronic illnesses resulting from it. The growing evidence, coupled with the anecdotal stories, strongly support the positive benefits of the anti-inflammatory diet. Are you experiencing mild inflammation? Do you just want to take positive steps toward improving your health? Then look into the anti-inflammatory diet and see if it will work for you.

The meat of this book has been the anti-inflammatory diet. We sincerely hope that the information provided will help you make the best decisions for yourself. There is a huge world out there full of vegan and vegetarian food. Go out there and enjoy it. Thank you for reading this Book.

Conclusion

Thank you for making it to the end of *Anti-Inflammatory Diet for Beginners*. Let's hope it was informative and able to provide you with all of the tools you need to achieve your goals whatever it is that they may be. This book provided a lot of information about a nutritious diet that will provide many health benefits and may even save someone's life. It is up to you if you would like to follow it in order to live a healthier lifestyle to prevent chronic illnesses and have a better quality of life. Quality of life is what we are promoting the most with the anti-inflammatory diet.

The next step is to start using the information presented in this book and begin incorporating it into your everyday life. We spoke extensively in this eBook about the inflammatory disease and how to prevent or resolve it with a proper diet. The anti-inflammatory diet will provide you with nutritious and delicious meals. Include it in your own meal prep and create a daily, weekly, or monthly meal schedule so you can stay ahead of the game. Avoiding serious health consequences is an important part of living a long and productive life. A proper diet is instrumental in creating that life for all of us. We know that we were oftentimes blunt when going over information in this book. But we want to make sure people understand the risks of inflammatory disease and the importance of an anti-inflammatory diet.

If you write it down, you are more likely to do it. You are more likely to do something if you get some type of enjoyment out of it. Enjoy it then. Try the recipes in this book, get creative with your own recipes, do even more research, and just have fun eating great food. It may seem like a chore at first. Change is never easy, but oftentimes, it is for the better, especially with matters regarding our health. Chronic inflammatory disease is no laughing matter. It is a disease that causes much suffering and can lead to many health problems down the line. Avoid these at all costs by sticking to an anti-inflammatory diet. The benefits will be tremendous.

Finally, if you found this book useful in any way, a review on Amazon is always appreciated.

Description

If you want to learn how to significantly improve your health and well-being and fight inflammatory disease simply by changing your eating habits, then keep reading and you will be amazed by what new information you learn!

We Are Here to Answer Some of Your Most Important Questions.

- Do you want to get healthy and wellness from an anti-inflammatory diet?
- Do you want to know what inflammation and inflammatory disease are?
- Do you want to know how to combat prolonged inflammation simply by changing your eating habits?
- Do you want to learn how you can avoid years of joint pain and muscle stiffness?
- Do you want to increase your energy levels?
- Do you want to increase your mood?
- Do you want to learn how to avoid chronic illnesses?
- Do you want to learn about delicious vegan and vegetarian meal plans?
- Do you want to learn how you can travel and still eat healthily?
- Do you want to improve your overall quality of life?

Imagine waking up every morning and barely being able to get out of bed. Your morning consists of taking multiple medications for various illnesses that you have. You head to work and whatever breaks you can get are spent making appointments for various doctors that you have to see on a regular basis. This is your life every day, filled with chronic pain, chronic illnesses, and being at the mercy of poor health and pharmaceuticals. Now, imagine that you can avoid all of this and have a significantly better quality of life. With a quality, anti-inflammatory diet, chronic illnesses like heart disease, kidney failure, stroke, and even cancer can be avoided. Chronic Inflammation can lead to a wealth of health problems. Proper eating habits can reduce and even prevent these problems from occurring and give you a lifestyle you will enjoy. This is not hyperbole; it is a reality.

By reading this book, you will obtain the knowledge you need to:

- Understand the inflammatory process and inflammatory disease.
- Understand the further health risks of prolonged, untreated inflammatory disease.
- Avoid or correct prolonged inflammation.
- Avoid chronic pain and many serious illnesses.
- Incorporate the inflammatory diet into your everyday life.

- Learn about delicious meal plans that follow the anti-inflammatory diet.
- Learn about meal plans from all over the world in case you love to travel.

Ready to learn more about the anti-inflammatory diet and its amazing benefits? Everyone can truly enjoy and get something out of this book.

- This book is for you if you are not currently on a healthy diet plan.
- This book is for you if you suffer from chronic pain and illness.
- This book is for you if you are relatively healthy but still want to learn more about diet and avoiding chronic disease.
- This book has something new for everybody, no matter what age, to learn because we touch on so many topics related to the anti-inflammatory diet.

Get this book today and discover the best anti-inflammatory foods! Would you like to know more? Go to the top of this page and click Buy Now!

CPSIA information can be obtained
at www.ICGtesting.com
Printed in the USA
LVHW100737150121
676498LV00025B/480

9 781801 232746